RBT Study Guide

By Newstone Test Prep

Table of Contents

****The exam simulator instructions, additional tests and other files can be downloaded by using the QR code located on the last page of this book.**

If the QR code does not work for you, please contact us at info@newstonetestprep.com and mention the title of this book.

Introduction to the BCBA Examination

About the Behavior Analyst Certification Board

For more than 20 years, the Behavior Analyst Certification Board, Inc. (BCBA) has been the industry pioneer in behavior analyst certification.

The BCBA was founded in 1998 to meet the demands for credentials recognized by behavior analyzers, governments and users of behavior-analytic services.

It aims to systematically define, promote and disseminate professional standards of practice to safeguard consumers of behavior-analytic services.

Eligibility Requirements

You must fulfill specific eligibility conditions and pass the RBT licensing exam to obtain the Registered Behavior Technician certification.

The specifications were put in place to guarantee that RBTs in entry-level positions have the knowledge, skills and aptitude required to provide behavior analysis services under the guidance of a competent supervisor.

Applicants must:

- Be over the age of 18
- Not have any criminal history
- Have a high school diploma or equivalent
- Complete 40 hours of training
- Satisfactorily finish an RBT preliminary competency test

General Rules for Taking the Examination at a Pearson VUE Testing Center

- To give yourself enough time to check in, you should arrive at the testing facility around 30 minutes before your scheduled exam time. Security precautions in this process include photographing and collecting an email signature from each candidate. You will not be allowed into the testing room 30 minutes after the test begins.

- To enter the examination area, you must present TWO kinds of current and genuine identification. Moreover, your first and last names must appear on both forms of identification as they appear on your BCBA account.
- You are not allowed to bring any of the following into the examination area: cameras, phones, recording equipment, beepers, other electronic devices, notes or reference materials, briefcases, bags, portfolios or handbags. Lockers are available at all examination locations for storing personal belongings.
- If you go to the bathroom during the examination, you will have your palms scanned both when you leave and return. You are not permitted to access anything kept in a locker during breaks, including phones, electronics or notes. However, you may access food, liquids and medications during breaks.
- Testing facilities do not have designated smoking areas.
- During the exam, you cannot ask any questions regarding the exam's subject matter. Please read all instructions attentively and pay close attention to what test center staff members say.

Section 1: Measurement

Chapter 1: Data Collection – Continuous and Discontinuous Measurements

As an RBT, it is vital to be knowledgeable about data collection so you can help treat and observe clients. This includes preparing for data collection, its importance, what happens when data is not measured and what data collection helps determine.

It also means conducting a task analysis of data, which includes crucial steps that need to be taken before beginning data collection, such as eliminating any distractions. However, you cannot just begin collecting data without any preparation. You have to find out which measurement procedure best fits your needs before you start.

So, specific methods and procedures are necessary for RBTs. They are covered below.

Preparing for Data Collection

Data collection is a necessary skill to learn when studying applied behavior analysis because employment agencies require data collection, both in digital and paper form. The data records ensure correct client analysis. If data is not adequately measured, it places technicians at a disadvantage and leaves them without the information needed to treat their clients.

From the technician's perspective, it is essential to collect data because data helps record any positive progress made by clients and can allow RBTs to observe new behaviors not previously seen. These observations may help RBTs conclude if the therapy is having a negative or positive impact.

Data collection is an excellent way of comparing different observations to improve the reliability of the results and ensure a client's history is documented and reflected on at a later date in order to provide the best support.

For example, recording and observing through the frequency method allows technicians to make conclusions about specific behavior, how likely it is to occur and if the occurrence may be higher or lower than the average. The analysis involved in measuring clients' behavior provides technicians with a range of information they can use to correctly and accurately assess their clients.

Task Analysis of Data Collection

The six steps below detail the task analysis of data collection:

Determine the Type of Behavior

For practical task analysis, it is essential to determine the type of behavior you are collecting data about. Different behaviors require different measures to provide the most valid result.

Find the Best Data Collection Method

RBTs are required to determine the best data collection method at this stage. They must make a decision based on specific clients and what they want to accomplish with them.

For example, when determining how long a specific action or behavior lasts, technicians may choose continuous measuring methods.

However, technicians must keep this rule in mind: they must always choose the most efficient data collection method. The method should not take too long, must provide accurate results and should not stress the client.

Gather the Materials Needed

It is vital to create an environment in which data collection is accessible. So, technicians must gather all necessary materials to proceed with data collection, including a pen, paper, timer, Excel sheet, data collection sheet, clipboard or any other needed materials.

The material required is specific to the data collection method. For example, when recording observations, technicians may use a pen and paper.

Enter Identifying Information

The next step is to fill out a form with the client's identifying information, such as name, date of birth, date and time of observation, diagnosis and the specific behavior or skill currently under observation.

The form will help RBTs analyze their clients more efficiently and determine the possible reasons for their behaviors. If RBTs do not have access to a standard form, they should write clients' identifying information in a notebook.

Eliminate Distractions

To ensure a reliable assessment and analysis, technicians must eliminate extraneous variables and control the environment. An example of an extraneous variable is a noisy room.

The assessment environment should be free of distractions that may impact clients and technicians. A controlled environment must be maintained to ensure clients are not disturbed or distracted when displaying the target behavior and the apparent reason for it.

Additionally, a controlled environment will help RBTs remain focused, providing a more reliable result.

Start Data Collection

After RBTs have completed all the steps, they have everything they need to begin data collection. They must then choose a suitable method to continue their data collection. The method chosen can depend on a range of reasons, such as the client's needs and the resources available.

For example, suppose the target behavior being observed is long term or permanent and the observer can invest limited time into the observation. In that case, the RBT may choose to use permanent-product recording features.

Continuous Measurement Procedures

Continuous measurement procedures record every instance of behavioral occurrence during a day or session. They are called continuous because they record every instance and are usually conducted over a short period of time.

Some examples of continuous measurement procedures include:

Frequency

Frequency consists of counting how many times an event occurs. When finding the frequency, the observer counts how often an event occurs.

For example, Sara threw a tantrum 10 times yesterday. The frequency is 10. It is simply the number or count of a specific behavior. Similarly, if Daniel stopped himself from getting angry six times during the week, then the frequency is six.

Duration

Duration is a method used to measure the length of time a behavior occurs. A timer may be used when recording duration data.

An observer will start the timer when a specific behavior occurs and stop it when it ends. The RBT will note down the duration on paper or an electronic document.

For example, if Sarah throws a tantrum, the RBT observing her may start a timer when she begins screaming and stop it when her fit ends. Noting how long a behavior lasts will help the RBT determine when it begins to decrease during later stages of the therapy.

Latency

Latency is the time between the beginning of a stimulus and the beginning of a response, or between the instruction and the beginning of a response.

For example, an observer says, “Stand up,” and starts a timer. The client takes three seconds to stand up and the timer stops. The latency is three seconds. Latency is directly related to inter-response time.

IRT

Inter-response time (IRT) is the duration of time between two responses. It is essential that the two responses be in the same response class.

To put it simply, IRT is the time between the end of one response and the start of another similar response.

Although IRT can initially seem confusing, it is simply the time between two responses.

Let's look at an example.

Daniel nods at 9:23 a.m. and asks a question at 9:25 after listening to some advice. During these two time points, Daniel does not provide any other response to his observer. Thus, the IRT duration is two minutes.

Discontinuous Measurement Procedures

Discontinuous measurement procedures record a sample of behavior during an observation.

However, some instances in discontinuous measurement procedures may not be recorded or detected, as every occurrence may not be observed.

Whole Interval Recording

Whole interval recording is when the behavior occurs for the whole interval set before the recording. The behavior is recorded as occurring only if it happens throughout an entire predetermined interval—typically ranging from 5 to 15 seconds.

At the end of every interval, the RBT records if the behavior occurred throughout. In whole interval recording, the behavior may be underestimated due to a timer and could possibly lead to an inaccurate reading.

An example is if the client screamed for the entire 10-second interval set by the observer.

Partial Interval Recording

In a partial interval recording, behavior is recorded as reoccurring if it happens at least once during the preset interval. This means that observation and recording are partial and do not occur throughout the interval.

Simply put, a partial interval recording is a time sampling procedure in which the observation period may be divided into a series of brief time intervals, usually ranging from 5 to 10 seconds.

In partial interval recording, it is not necessary to note how often a specific behavior occurs or the duration of the behavior. The observer is required to record the behavior only if it occurred more than once or happened in the predetermined time intervals.

For example, if Sabrina tries to interrupt the observer twice during a 10-minute preset interval, a partial interval recording occurs.

Momentary Time Sampling

Momentary time sampling records if behavior occurred at one particular moment. Similar to a whole and partial interval recording, the sampling has a predetermined time frame. The behavior is noted or recorded only if it occurs when the predetermined time interval ends.

For example, if an RBT observes crying behavior for five seconds, he or she will record a plus (+) if the crying occurred at the end of the five seconds or a minus (-) if the crying did not occur or happen at the end of the interval. The absence of crying is not officially recorded because it does not prove to be of any help in observing the targeted behavior.

Permanent-Product Recording Features

Permanent-product recording features measure the end product of a specific behavior by observing its effect on the environment. It does not require the direct observation of a specific or target behavior.

Since direct observation is not required, this method is more time efficient than continuous and discontinuous methods of measuring data. For example, a teacher provides a percentage grade on the correct answers on a math test even if the teacher did not witness the student attempting all the questions. The concern may be only with the result.

The method is suitable when the behavior being looked at results in a permanent or lasting outcome, is not short-lived or temporary, or there is not enough time to conduct behavioral observations.

Chapter 2: Measuring End Products, Graphs and Behaviors

Measuring the end product of behavior is vital to RBT training because it helps provide different methods for measuring behavior. So, as an RBT, you may be expected to know the basics of analyzing and recording data efficiently, such as with the help of different graphs.

Different graphs have different strengths. For example, a bar chart may not be suitable for plotting information gathered by continuous measurements, such as duration, because the gathered information in this data measurement depends on time. So, using a line graph to plot the data may be appropriate.

Permanent-Product Recording

Permanent-product recording procedures are standard in behaviors with long-lasting or permanent effects. They are concerned with the end product instead of the process of how the result was obtained. This is important to note, as discontinuous and continuous methods—like rate, frequency, duration and whole interval periods—consider and observe the entire process.

Thus, to implement permanent-product recording procedures, the RBT must focus on measuring the end product of an observation rather than the process.

Unfortunately, permanent-product recording may be difficult to follow because of the time requirement. So, the simplest way to measure permanent-product recording features is by first organizing what is being measured and dividing it into sections, such as:

1. The date when the permanent product was completed. This refers to the actual date or, in some instances, the time when the specific behavior was finished being observed or successfully treated. This can help establish a timeline for the behavior in question.
2. The label or name of the permanent product. It is essential to name the behavior being observed—for example, aggression—and whether it is seen as unfavorable in the technician's observation.

3. The number of times (frequency) the target behavior occurred. For example, if Sara hit her sister four times, the frequency would then be four.
4. The number of opportunities in which the behavior could have occurred. The client's environment significantly impacts how likely the target emotion is to occur. It can be observed and noted how often the client had the opportunity to act on the target behavior being studied.
5. The total number of times the conduct or target behavior occurred.

The following data table can account for the different values and possible progress in a client's behavior. The information in the table is then added to a graph.

Date	**Permanent-Product Label**	**Number of Times Behavior Occurred**	**Number of Opportunities**	**Total % of Times Behavior Occurred**
9/4	Homework Section 1	8	10	(8/10) x 100 = 80
9/5	Homework Section 2	14	20	(14/20) x 100 = 70
9/6	Homework Section 3	5	20	(5/15) x 100 = 25

In this example, the behavior is the number of questions answered correctly in a homework assignment, and the permanent product would be the homework assignments turned in. The percentages 80%, 70% and 25% may then be added to a graph, in addition to the respective permanent product label.

When the technician has recorded all the information mentioned above, the next step is to choose the graph method for plotting the data. A bar graph may be the most suitable method when measuring end products in permanent-product recording features, as the information can be shown efficiently.

Graphs Used in Data Collection and How to Enter Data into Charts

Various graphs are used in data collection. Each graph must have a data table (as shown above) to ensure the information is organized and easily plotted. The data table improves efficiency and will be required when measuring data in any session.

Using graphed data is crucial, as it helps communicate information about the observation, shows a relationship or link between the dependent and independent variables and supports the data-based instructional decision-making process.

The following are some types of graphs:

Bar Chart

If a comparison needs to be made between different values in the same subject, a bar chart is one of the best options.

Using a bar chart, the RBT can visually represent the progress made in a client's behavior and whether any significant changes need to be investigated to ensure the client is given the best possible help.

After entering all client data into the table, the RBT can then input the critical values into the bar chart. Any new data can also be easily entered by creating another set of bars or a singular bar to highlight any differences in behavior.

An example of a data collection bar chart is shown below:

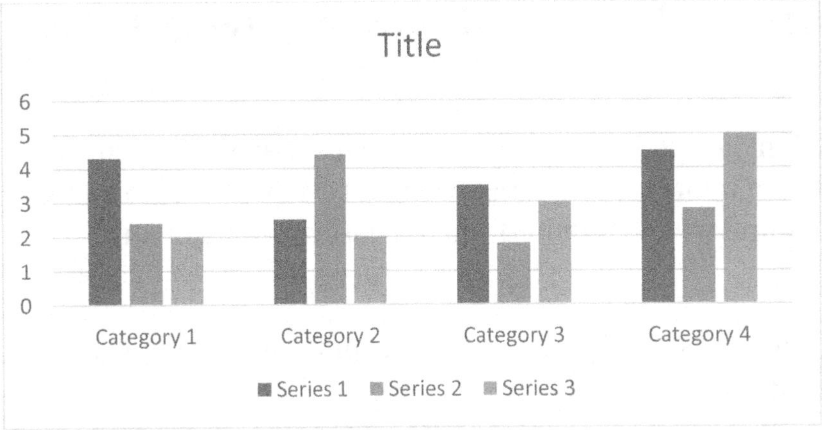

Pie Chart

In a pie chart, data must first be recorded in the data table and then entered into the pie chart.

A pie chart is ideal for categorizing data, as every segment in the graph represents a specific category. It may also be suitable for describing multiple target behaviors and comparing them.

The example below provides a possible way of entering data into a pie chart:

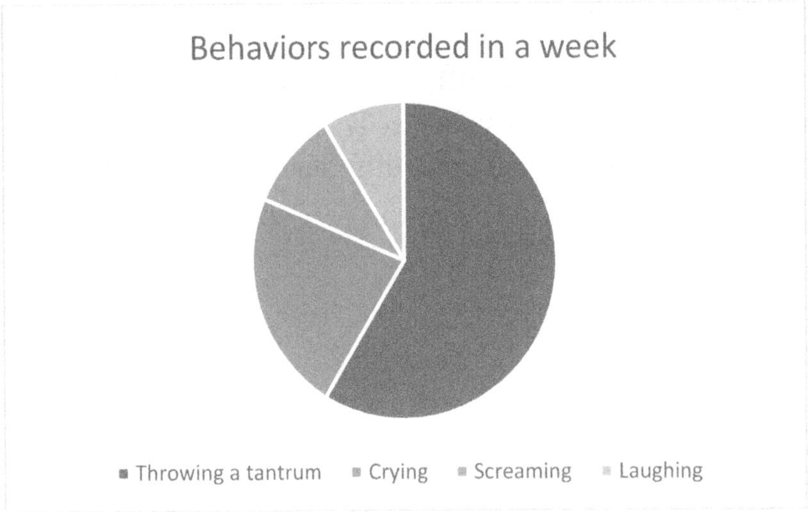

Line Graph

A line graph is ideal for showing change—long or short—over time. It can also be easily edited to enter more information, which can be done by adding the next point.

In a line graph, points are connected with the help of straight lines and are used when multiple sets of information need to be compared.

Unlike a bar or pie chart, a line graph is based on time and the progression or regression of behavior during the selected period. The x-axis in a line graph is usually based on a period. In contrast, the measure or quantity of behavior may be on the y-axis.

For example, Johnny throws a tantrum two times in five minutes. The quantity is two and the time is five minutes. In the line graph, the dependent variable is the client's behavior and the independent variable is the duration.

The slope of a line in the line graph is critical. It compares the depth of change between two consecutive points in the chart. The steeper the slope of a line, the larger the difference between the x-axis and y-axis.

Use Measurable and Observable Terms to Describe Behavior and the Environment

Behavior can be defined as observable and measurable actions in physical functions. Simply put, it is anything that can be heard or seen. In behavioral science, emotions or feelings are not categorized as behaviors.

Although they may be subjective terms, it is essential to define specific behaviors as either "good" or "bad" when measuring them. This helps determine the progress or regression in a particular set of behaviors. For example, aggressive behavior may be labeled as harmful or bad and peaceful or happy behavior may be labeled as good, depending on what the technician is measuring and the observation's aim.

It is essential to consider the function when it comes to behavior. In fact, the reason a behavior occurred is necessary to note in RBT training. As a technician, it is vital not to provide a conclusion and instead provide evidence. For example, "Sara was aggressive" is not an acceptable analysis. Instead, "Sara hit her sister five times because she was angry" gives a reason for Sara's behavior instead of a conclusion. An acceptable analysis is also important because aggressive behavior can be measured quantitatively.

The environment is anything perceived through the senses. So, it is essential to be specific with the definitions of behavior and environment; this data is precise and can be quickly understood by a new technician if required. The environment is essential when identifying the function of behavior; it may explain specific behavior or provide crucial context to the situation.

As an RBT, it is crucial to consider changes in the recorded target behavior. Any progress or decline must be noted so you can check back in your notes and determine if the therapy currently taking place is suitable for your client. If it is not, you may choose to follow a different therapy.

Therapy progress can be easily documented using graphs, providing fellow technicians or learners with a chance to learn from a particular case.

Section 2: Assessment

Chapter 3: Preference, Individualized and Functional Assessments

Preference Assessment

Preference assessment in applied behavior analysis (ABA) can be described as a guiding tool RBTs use to reinforce their clients. It is conducted to increase the probability of positive behavior being performed in the future.

Simply put, a preference assessment tells what will act as a motivation for a client and at what specific point in time.

When a client is engaging in appropriate behavior, the reinforcer will provide the client with something that increases the chances of this response often occurring in the future.

So, with the help of a preference assessment, the RBT can decide which stimuli will be suitable for the client and under what circumstances.

Importance of Preference Assessments

Preference assessments are necessary to ensure the maximum level of skill acquisition programs. This is done by ensuring the highest preferred stimuli can be used as potential reinforcers for new skills.

The highest select items used as reinforcers can also help reduce inappropriate behavior, which is possible through automatic positive reinforcement. For example, if a client screams at the RBT, the technician may positively convey to the client that these actions are not right and reinforce the need for patience.

While assessment preferences are used to identify potential reinforcers for the client, it is not confirmed whether the chosen reinforcer will increase positive behavior in a client or not. It is confirmed only when the reinforcer is used.

So, to accurately determine whether a reinforcer can motivate the client, the RBT must ask the client a few questions.

The RBT can start by asking clients about their preferences. Stakeholders—like parents, caregivers and teachers—can also be asked about clients' preferences. Open-ended questions, multiple-choice format or rank-ordering are some ways RBTs can proceed with this method.

Types of Preference Assessments

From systematic data collection to casual questions, there are many ways to conduct preference assessments. A few assessment types are described below.

Multiple Stimulus with Replacement

The multiple stimulus with replacement assessment presents a variety of stimuli and clients select the one they want the most. The chosen stimulus remains and all other incentives are replaced with new stimuli.

The assessment is appropriate for clients who can select their preferred stimuli from an array of items. It can also be appropriate for children who do not engage in challenging behavior when their preferred toy is taken away. It is the most suitable way of treating clients who engage in problem behavior when preferred toys are taken away from them.

When using this assessment technique, an RBT places an array of items in front of the child. These items usually include toys or food. The child chooses one item from the array. As soon as one item is taken or consumed, the RBT takes the other items and replaces them. A trial happens each time new items are presented. The trials are repeated until a set number of trials is achieved or until the child refuses to choose any more items.

Multiple Stimulus Without Replacement

A multiple stimulus without replacement assessment is most suitable for children who do not engage in problem behavior when a preferred toy is taken away. It is the quickest, most accurate way for children with prerequisite skills.

The RBT places an array of items in front of the client. There is no set number of items to be used in the array, but six to eight items are a good amount. The client then chooses a preferred item one by one. The RBT marks and records the order in which the client selects the items. The technician's notes show the most preferred to the least preferred items.

Several things are to be considered when recording the results of this method. One of these is the amount of time it took for the client to make a decision, which shows what items the client prefers the most and the least.

Paired Stimulus

A paired-stimulus preference assessment is appropriate for clients who can choose a preferred item from one or two arrays of chosen highly selected items and low-preferred items.

The best method for assessing the client's preference is by pairing a highly preferred item and a low-preferred item side by side and observing the client's reaction.

The thing to focus on here is whether the client consistently chooses the highly preferred item over the low-preferred item. This method, however, should not be used if the client has trouble choosing one item over another.

Single Stimulus

A single-stimulus preference assessment is best for clients who cannot choose between highly preferred and low-preferred items and clients engaging in challenging behavior when preferred toys are taken away from them. This is because, in this method, clients can engage with preferred items until they finally stop, get tired or give the items up.

However, this method takes time. So, it might not be suitable if a quick assessment is required.

Free-Operant Observations

The free-operant method is suitable for all clients. However, it is most appropriate for clients who engage in challenging behavior when items are taken away from them. It can be done regularly in a simple classroom setting or be scheduled during a time when the client has the opportunity to choose among many different items or activities.

Reinforcement is a crucial part of being an effective RBT. Even though there are a variety of preference assessment procedures that have shown to be effective in research, learners showing what they want is most effective in identifying and choosing preferred items as reinforcements.

Individualized Assessments

Individualized assessments refer to the process of gathering information about a particular client to determine what the person's needs are. Assessment is conducted to determine a client's skills, the amount of time of services a client requires and the progress the individual makes.

Assessment methods must be conducted based on the individual client. One of the first things to keep in mind or remember is the client's age. Some assessment methods are appropriate for toddlers and children, while others are appropriate for adults. Similarly, some assessment methods focus on learning skills in school, while some focus on language skills.

So, abilities, skills, age and language are factors that need to be considered before the assessment procedure is taken forward.

For example, if a client's skills need to be assessed, a preference assessment method might not be appropriate. Individualized assessments can come in various forms, including formal, informal, indirect and direct. RBTs can choose any of these to test their clients' skills.

It is essential to conduct assessments frequently to track a client's progress. Individualized assessments make it easier for the BCBA to determine what to focus on during intervention planning. Aside from that, an individualized assessment provides a baseline for a client analysis.

Assessments also give the client's parents, teachers and caregivers a clear understanding of the client's skill level. This way, everyone involved with the client can be on the same page.

Assessment of Social Competency

An assessment of social competency can be necessary for multiple reasons. The most common causes include:

- Poor social skills
- Difficulty making eye contact
- Struggling with classroom demands
- Difficulty making friends or communicating.

This assessment aims to improve clients' social skills and identify the social challenges they face.

Curriculum-Based Assessment

A curriculum-based assessment shows changes in progress. The assessment directly assesses targeted skills in essential areas or topics.

Functional Behavior Assessment

The functional behavioral assessment (FBA) aims to identify the cause of challenging behavior in a client and find a possible solution for it.

The FBA assessment involves identifying challenging behavior, hypothesizing its function and guiding the development of a treatment plan. Even though all assessment methods have the same purpose, the FBA's specific goal is to identify the purpose of the function of a behavior.

Some of the typical functions of behavior include:

1. Attention seeking
2. Seeking access to things
3. Automatic reinforcement
4. Escape

There are different kinds of FBAs.

Indirect Functional Assessment

The indirect functional assessment involves gathering information about the client from people who spend the maximum amount of time with him or her. This can consist of parents, teachers, caregivers, etc.

Indirect functional methods can include rating scales, questionnaires and interviews. The goal is to gather enough information to analyze the reasons for a client's behavior.

For instance, giving clients a questionnaire to examine their feelings would be an example of an indirect functional assessment.

Direct Functional Assessment

The direct functional assessment involves direct observation of the client in the individual's natural environment. The sessions can also include the client's parents, teachers or caregivers.

One way of conducting a direct assessment is a time chart. A mark is made on the time and day of the behavior. This helps determine the time when a particular behavior occurs. It also becomes much easier to identify the reason behind it.

For example, if a child usually engages in a challenging behavior at 7:00 p.m., it will be marked on the time chart. The mark can help identify the events or reasons that make the child engage in such behavior. The reasons could involve activities the child does not like, such as bath time or brushing teeth.

ABC Data Collection

ABC data collection is a tool used in ABA for recording behaviors. It can be used by RBTs, teachers, parents and caregivers for a variety of reasons, such as assessing behavior, identifying the behavior's function, tracking a client's progress and documenting behavior tendencies.

How Does ABC Data Collection Work?

ABC data collection tool is divided into three parts:

1. **The Antecedent**

The antecedent is the actions, circumstances and events before a behavior. For example, a child is asked to do something like pick up a piece of paper from the ground.

2. **The Behavior**

The behavior is the result of the antecedent. For example, the same child will not pick up the paper but instead will scream and shout when asked to do so.

3. **The Consequence**

The consequence is the child watching the RBT picking up other items from the ground while asking the child to pick up the paper again.

Several things must be kept in mind during this procedure. First, it is essential to record observations in a way that makes them more accessible for others to understand. Similarly, the observations should be completely subjective and based on what is seen rather than what the observer felt.

Other than this, when the data is collected completely, the ABC team might, in some cases, collaborate with the BCBA to help the client transition from challenging to appropriate behavior.

ABC data collection is just one tool the RBT uses to assist in understanding a client's behavior.

Section 3: Skill Acquisition

Chapter 4: Looking into Written Skill Acquisition

In this chapter, we look into written skill acquisition. First, we will cover what is meant by written skill acquisition and discuss the importance of data behavior analysis to determine how students gain proficiency in transferrable abilities.

Next, we will cover the essential components of a written skill acquisition plan that includes a description of the target behavior/skill, material needed to teach the skill, strategies to teach the skill and the consequences for correct and incorrect answers.

Lastly, we will cover strategies needed to prepare for a written skill acquisition plan, including the conditions necessary to hold a session with a client.

What Is Written Skill Acquisition?

A skill acquisition plan is a written plan prepared by a behavior analyst that includes information on behavior programming to teach specific skills.

It must include:

- A description of the target skill being taught
- The required teaching materials
- The prompting strategies to be used
- The consequences for responding correctly or incorrectly
- A mastery criterion
- Reinforcement techniques
- A generalization and maintenance plan

The Importance of Data

Nearly every significant feature of any professional athlete is routinely evaluated, analyzed and documented. This is done so the players may assess if they are growing better, remaining stagnant or becoming worse by receiving immediate and accurate feedback on their performance. The same is true for the autistic students you may work with.

RBTs are in charge of continuously evaluating learners' development. They keep track of a range of information about clients' behavior and assess if they are growing better, remaining stagnant or becoming worse by receiving immediate and accurate feedback on their performance.

The collected data can be analyzed to identify relevant response patterns, such as increases or decreases in target behaviors. Data is critical in determining the effectiveness of instructional methods and when to start teaching new skills or behaviors. It is also used to decide when to change prompting strategies to promote student independence.

How Do Behavioral Analysts Use Data to Understand Human Behavior?

Behavioral analysts use a variety of data to understand human behavior. This is collected through surveys, interviews, observational data and demographics.

1. **Surveys** – They are used to collect data on human behavior. This data can include information on attitudes, beliefs and preferences.
2. **Interviews** – They are used to collect data about experiences, feelings and motivations.
3. **Observational Data** – This is used to understand human behavior. This data can include information about facial expressions, body language and how people interact with others.
4. **Demographic Data** – This is mostly used to understand human behavior. This data can include age, gender, ethnicity and socioeconomic status information.

Analysts can use the data collected to understand how people think, feel and behave. Their understanding can help individuals with mental health disorders as well as help businesses understand their customers' motivations and behaviors.

Behavioral analysts can use data to predict how people will behave in certain situations, which can be very helpful for businesses.

So, what do behavioral analysts do with all this data? Well, there are a few different applications. One is market research. By understanding consumer behavior, businesses can better target their products and services to specific audiences. Behavioral analysts can provide insights into how people make decisions, which can help inform government policymaking.

Finally, one of the most critical applications of behavioral data is in mental health. By understanding how people think and behave, clinicians can develop better treatments for mental health conditions.

Data Components Used by RBTs

For improvement, accurate measurement of the actual behavior is required. Information is necessary to show that participants' behavior has changed.

Applied interventions focus on behavior that can be measured (or reported). Measurement may include using the following types of data:

1. **Frequency Data** – How often a behavior occurs within a given time frame. The behavior must have a clear start and stop.
2. **Duration Data** – The length of time a behavior occurs. It specifies the time measurement.
3. **Partial Interval** – When the target behavior occurs for a part of a specified period.
4. **Whole Interval** – When the target behavior occurs for the entire duration of a specified period.
5. **Permanent Products** – The tangible outcomes of specific behaviors.
6. **Scatterplot** – Recording the occurrence of a particular behavior over an extended period. It indicates a pattern that may be related to the time of day, day of the week or event/activity associated with a particular time.

The Essential Components of a Written Skill Acquisition Plan

Behavior analysts working with individuals who have developmental disabilities often utilize a skill acquisition plan. This is a plan that helps RBTs teach new skills to individuals. Let's discuss how to prepare a written skill acquisition plan.

1. First, it is essential to have a clear understanding of the individual's current level of functioning. This will help identify what skills need to be taught.

2. Next, a task analysis should be conducted. This will involve breaking down the new skill into smaller, more manageable steps.

3. Once the task analysis is complete, a schedule should be created. This is a detailed plan of when each task step will be taught. Specific times must be mentioned.

4. Finally, it is crucial to select an appropriate reinforcement schedule because this will help motivate the individual to learn a new skill.

Moreover, the skill acquisition plan must be well written, easily followed and implemented. A well-written skill-acquisition strategy includes:

1. A description of the skill that needs to be acquired
2. An established standard for skill acquisition. (Establishing a baseline helps figure out a program's goal.)
3. A specific objective that shows the development of a skill. (Data enables the result of skill acquisition. Providers can evaluate if an activity or aim successfully teaches desired skills if a goal is clearly defined.)
4. A thorough description of the steps. The procedure that should be followed to achieve skill objectives is described by the ABA using a common prescriptive language:
    - Presentation – A method of teaching
    - Instructions – The desired response
    - SR +/- – Reinforcement and plan for reinforcement
    - Error correction (EC) – Correcting errors
5. Reactionary techniques to use when unwanted conduct or a delayed display of the skill occurs. (Targets for skill acquisition must always contain an error correction.)
6. Techniques for gathering and displaying data used to gauge the program's effectiveness
7. Methods to regularly review the information and situation
8. Strategies for skill upkeep and service termination. (A fading approach will be a part of a well-developed plan. It outlines how to reduce service hours correctly while maintaining therapeutic potential. This often happens after clients have reached their skill goals and behavior has reduced.)

Description of the Target Behavior/Skill

Behavior includes all the observable and measurable actions living organisms take. However, a target behavior is a reaction resembling the trainer's model and takes place within three seconds. It should specify what particular target response you are expecting from the client.

For example, if you are teaching a client with ASD (autism spectrum disorder) categories, in response to the instruction "Give me examples of a few colors," a correct answer on the part of the client might be "Red, yellow, blue."

A specific description of the behavior makes it easier to administer a treatment program consistently and specifies the reactions that should lead to positive reinforcement. A behavioral goal that is precisely defined must contain three necessary components:

1. A description of the circumstance under which the conduct will take place
2. A description of the desired behavior
3. A description of the requirements for success

Material Needed to Teach the Skill

The materials needed to support the learning results must be consistent with the teaching methods. Trained tutors, materials and technology are required to carry out a learning method.

The structure of the materials, how they should be used and whether or not they should all be included is based on each learner's needs.

Your skill acquisition plan should include a list of the specific instructional resources needed to complete the program. For instance, you will need bread, butter, ham and a knife if you are teaching an adult with ASD how to make a sandwich.

Strategies to Teach the Skill

For skill acquisition, there needs to be a learning strategy. A learning strategy is a set of organized activities that help students achieve their learning objectives. They should be the most effective activities to attain the desired result, whether they are learner- or teacher-centered. These strategies are ideally based on the learner's preferred learning style.

It is ideal for a learning plan to include various adult learning activities, such as self-directed learning, experiential learning and reflexivity, which work together to produce a comprehensive learning experience.

To define an action, learning techniques should be written using specific phrases like *review, identify, perform, describe, construct* and *apply*. These key terms are reflected in the exercises designed to increase the knowledge and abilities needed to direct the accomplishment of the learning outcome.

After the skill steps are defined, they are learned through a sequence of activities known as task analysis—a crucial teaching precept to support a learner's development from simple to advanced skill acquisition. Strategies involve multiple actions, suction reinforcement and prompting.

How to Choose the Strategy

Here's how to determine the plan strategy:

- Determine what happened in the previous session to understand where to begin.
- Choose which skill acquisition procedures will be completed during the session.
- Prepare the materials needed for the skill acquisition procedure (including data collection materials).

The procedures that RBTs use include:

- Discrete-trial teaching (DTT)
- Naturalistic teaching
- Pivotal response therapy
- Token economy
- Contingent observation

Most learners can benefit from a combination of DTT and naturalistic teaching. You can switch back and forth between the two to avoid boredom and provide the learner with transition flexibility.

Consequences for Correct and Incorrect Answers

A trainer may use reinforcement as a created contingency to promote behavior modification or skill development. Reinforcement occurs when a stimulus modification happens right after a response, increasing the likelihood that comparable situations will lead to more of the same behavior in the future.

Contingent reinforcement is the use of reinforcers conditional on a specific behavior. It is a technique that could be considered the foundation of ABA because it allows an RBT to reinforce a particular beneficial behavior while avoiding reinforcing undesirable behaviors.

In contrast, noncontingent reinforcement is primarily ineffective in cases of incorrect answers. This affects behavior patterns, but usually not in a way that can be controlled. Helplessness is the most common response. However, in some cases, it is used to condition a reaction to certain implicit rewards that would otherwise contribute to fixation and inappropriate behavior.

A child with autism who has meltdowns in class to get the teacher's attention, for example, may instead be given that attention at intervals unassociated with the tantrums. This lessens the link between the two and may result in less harmful behavior.

In cases of incorrect answers, prompting may occur. A prompt appears when an individual (typically the client) receives assistance completing an activity or exhibiting a specific behavior. A prompt in ABA helps learners achieve their treatment goals.

RBTs should also consider prompt fading, which means how they'll lower the prompts over time to ensure that learners achieve as much independence as possible.

A stimulus prompt is a cue that draws attention to the discriminative stimulus (SD) for the intended behavior. For instance, to encourage someone to pick a box, you may choose a huge box with a bold color.

In contrast, stimulus shaping is the gradual alteration of the stimulus's physical characteristics, such as making the container smaller and of different colors over time.

A stimulus that helps the subject generate the proper reaction is known as a cue. Response cues can be administered orally, by modeling or physically. It is not a prompt if the response is incorrect.

Reinforcement Strategies

The term *reinforcement* in ABA or any other behavioral therapy refers to giving support or cues to encourage the application of a particular skill. For example, if you are teaching a child to ask for candy, after the client says, "Candy, please," or "I want candy," you always give the child candy.

Reinforcement encourages clients to perform a task until they learn how and when to do it. Successful strategies also provide a task development timetable and realistic challenges to overcome. The goal is for the client to eventually perform the skill independently in the proper conditions without needing to be prompted.

However, the strategy may or may not specify which reinforcers should be used. This is because reinforcers for most skill acquisition plans should be changed regularly, depending on the learner's preferences.

Types of Reinforcements

There are several types of reinforcement:

- **Conditioned Reinforcement** – The phrase *conditioned reinforcement* refers to reinforcement enhanced by the presence of another reinforcer, such as toys, money, praise, grades, awards, tokens, etc.
- **Unconditioned Reinforcement** – Reinforcements that do not need training or conditioning are referred to as *unconditioned reinforcements*. Examples of unconditioned reinforcers include food, drink, painkillers and physical attention.

- **Intermittent Reinforcement** – *Intermittent reinforcement* plans produce reinforcement only when specific instances of the behavior occur, in contrast to continuous reinforcement schedules, which offer reinforcement for every incidence of the behavior. According to research, intermittent programs work better than continuous schedules at getting higher response rates.

Positive vs. Negative Reinforcements

Positive reinforcement means a consequence is added as a result of an action. For example, giving a child access to a favorite toy after solving a puzzle.

Remember, positive reinforcements are not only rewards; they just mean that an action has a consequence of reinforcing specific behavior. At the same time, a negative reinforcement means the consequence is removed. For example, an adult removes the punishment of extra homework because the child performed well at school.

Mastery Criteria

Behavioral practitioners and researchers often define skill acquisition as meeting specific mastery criteria.

A mastery criterion based on accuracy is linked to various factors, like the performance level (such as a particular percentage of accurate answers) and the number of observations required to reach this level (such as numerous sessions or a single-day session).

For example, if a client achieves at least 90% accuracy in identifying body parts with at least two different technicians on two days, we can say that those targets have been mastered with that particular instruction. Most are above the 80% mark. Some BCBAs prefer 90% or higher on all three days.

Maintenance

Maintenance is a learner's ability to demonstrate previously acquired skills over time and over durations in which reinforcement has shrunk below the level at which the skill was first taught.

Contingencies of Reinforcement

A contingency might be a reward or a penalty once an individual or group exhibits a behavior. In simpler words, a naturally occurring contingency is anything that happens as a natural consequence without the involvement of behavior analysts.

An example of this is pushing the snooze button. That makes you late for work and stops you from having breakfast at home. The naturally occurring default for pressing the snooze button is not having access to breakfast.

Behavior is strengthened by the process of reinforcement, which is a critical concept in behavior therapy. Schedules of reinforcement relate to how and when consequences for conduct are delivered. However, there are several types of schedules of reinforcement, such as:

- Fixed ratio (FR)
- Fixed interval (FI)
- Variable ratio (VR)
- Variable interval (VI)

When a reinforcement constantly occurs after the same number of responses, this is known as a fixed ratio. It is sometimes referred to as a fixed-time schedule because the amount of time dedicated to each reinforcer is constant.

Similarly, reinforcement is always supplied after a predetermined period with fixed-interval schedules. Variable ratio and variable interval refer to situations where the number of reinforcements necessary or the amount of time before reinforcement varies irregularly.

Example of Schedules of Reinforcement in Action

a. **Fixed Ratio**

- **FR1** – Every bite of broccoli results in a bite of French fries.
- **FR2** – Every two bites of broccoli result in a bite of French fries.

b. **Variable Ratio**

- **VR3** – On average, every three bites of broccoli results in a bite of French fries.

c. **Fixed Interval**

- **FI5 minutes** – After Joline plays independently for at least five minutes, the RBT will play with Joline if she asks.

d. **Variable Interval**

- **VI5 minutes** – After Joline plays independently for between three and seven minutes (five minutes on average), the RBT will play with Joline if she asks.

In contingent reinforcement, a trainer may use reinforcement or punishment as a created contingency to promote behavior modification or skill development. Giving a child access to a favorite toy after solving a puzzle illustrates this.

Giving reinforcement regularly without regard to conduct is known as noncontingent reinforcement (NCR). By providing the reinforcer freely and without conditions, the goal is to decrease the undesirable behavior and lower the motivation to engage in it.

To create an abolishing operation (AO) and a scenario of reinforcement satiation, NCR manipulates motivating operations. If, for instance, it is determined the behavior is performed to obtain attention, we may attempt to diminish its occurrence by providing regular attention.

The reinforcement rate dropping to a naturally accessible level is an indiscriminate contingency. You need to lower the reinforcement rate to an indiscriminate contingency to test for generalization.

However, during generalization, the client should not require prompts or ongoing reinforcement; instead, the indiscriminate contingency should be sufficient to keep the behavior in place.

Chapter 5: Implementing Teaching Procedures

Discrete-Trial Teaching (DTT)

DTT is one of the most well-studied treatment and education procedures for teaching skills to ASD learners. It is a teaching method in which learning trials are presented in rapid succession, with each trial having a distinct beginning and end.

There are three sections in DTT:

1. The instructions
2. The learner's response
3. The reinforcer

In DTT, the reinforcer may be unrelated to the skills being taught. Prompting is used to help learners respond correctly and then is faded out. After that, the RBT initiates trials.

DTT is typically fast-paced, with the technician trying to maximize the number of trials while reducing the time the learner must wait between attempts.

DTT can take place in several ways, such as:

- Matching objects
- Essential learning responding (identifying labels of things or following simple instructions)
- Motor and vocal imitation
- Language skills involving action
- Features
- Functions
- Cause and effect
- Categories
- Academic skills, including letters, numbers, shapes and colors

Components of DTT

The essential components of a DTT session include:

- Mixing and varying targets between using SD and prompting
- Concise instructions and a clear definition of a correct response
- Some examples of SD

Let's look at DTT components in detail:

1. **Discriminative Stimulus**

A quick, precise instruction alerting the client to the work at hand serves as the SD. It helps the client connect a specific direction with a suitable response.

An example is if a technician asks a client, "What is this?" before asking the individual to name an object.

2. **The Prompt**

A prompt could be required to help the client come up with the right response. It could be conducted between the SD and the response.

The prompt occurs when the technician guides the client's conduct by demonstrating the appropriate response. For instance, if it seems like the client is having trouble, the trainer may tap the right object.

3. **Client's Response and Consequence**

The client may react to the stimulus correctly or incorrectly. The intended reaction should be defined clearly and precisely before the trial.

The result will change depending on whether the response is correct or incorrect:

- **Correct Response** – Positive reinforcement is given right away for a correct response. The reward is frequently shown to clients beforehand, so they know what they will get. Before each trial, the type and value of the award are specified. The reward could be in the form of verbal praise, food (like sweets) or a token from a behavioral modification system (e.g., a point that goes toward the overall score).
- **Incorrect Response** – When clients respond incorrectly during a DTT trial, they are corrected without any negative consequence. The trainer makes an effort to maintain impartiality. Both rewards and

penalties are absent. For example, a technician might indicate the correct response and remark, “Let’s give this another try.”

4. **Inter-Trial Period**

The final stage of DTT is the inter-trial period. This is the time frame that follows the outcome. This stage signals the conclusion of one trial and the beginning of another.

Usually, the inter-trial period lasts no more than five seconds. Its brevity helps keep the learning process ongoing.

Steps of Conducting Discrete-Trial Teaching

1. Deliver the instruction. For example, say: “Put fingers on your lips.” If it is a prompted trial, pair a prompt with the instruction. In this case, the technician should also put the finger on his or her lips.
2. Wait three seconds for the learner to respond.
   a. Reinforce immediately and enthusiastically if the learner responds correctly. For example: Puts the finger on lips.
   b. Implement a correction procedure if the learner responds incorrectly or does not respond. For example, you could repeat the instruction while providing an immediate full prompt to ensure the learner responds correctly with the following learning opportunity.
3. Quickly record data.
4. Regain the learner’s attention (if necessary) and present the next instruction.

Data Collection

Data on the outcomes of each trial is typically collected to track the client’s progress. For example, data on whether a client responded correctly, required a prompt or answered incorrectly may be collected in an individual discrete trial.

A client’s percentage rates and performance levels are calculated by adding correct and incorrect responses.

Naturalistic Teaching Procedures

Incidental teaching is a strategy that employs ABA principles to provide structured learning opportunities in the natural environment by leveraging the learner's natural interests and motivation. It is used for skills that do not necessarily have a clear beginning and end.

Incidental teaching is effective for skills that are supposed to naturally occur at any time. This method does not require direct instruction. It is especially beneficial to young children.

In incidental teaching, the RBT chooses the activity or situation in which the learning opportunities will occur based on the learner's lead. The trainer gets involved in an incidental teaching episode; he or she points to appropriate situations that happen naturally.

Strategies encourage the learner's responses when a trainer acknowledges a naturally occurring situation in which a learner is showing interest. Incidental teaching strategies are intended to increase motivation and generalization.

How to Employ Naturalistic Teaching Procedures

1. Set up the environment.
2. Involve the learner in the procedure in the designated environment.
3. Reinforce the response if the learner's initiative is already sufficient for reinforcement.
4. Prompt a response if the learner's initiative is insufficient for reinforcement.
5. Reinforce and fade the prompt over time if the learner correctly responds to it.
6. Make sure the environment is ready for another learning opportunity.

Although naturalistic teaching appears to be play, it should always include effective prompting and contingent reinforcement. If getting sweets is a strong reinforcer for the learners, you could use candy to teach them how to draw a square.

For example, Isaac works as a preschool teacher. He knows that William is fond of giraffes, but the child's language skills need improvement. During the lesson,

Isaac places a giraffe just out of reach (environment). William observes the giraffe and asks Isaac to bring it a bit closer, initiating communication with Isaac (response). Isaac compliments William and hands him the giraffe (reinforcement)

Let's look at another example.

Isaac is training another student, Suzanne, who loves the color red. He strategically puts a bright red pencil out of Suzanne's reach during a transitional phase (environment). Suzanne exhibits delayed communication by failing to request the pencil. Isaac shrugs at Suzanne, indicating he has no idea what she wants (prompt). Suzanne points to the pencil, which Isaac hands her as a reward (reinforcement). He also allows her to play her favorite song on his phone (to reinforce for another activity).

How to Optimize Learning Opportunities in the Natural Environment

Determine Learners' Interests

Determine the learner's current interests to increase engagement. Note which materials, actions and objects motivate the learner at any given time. The object of interest or activity of interest should be appropriate for the learner's developmental level.

Remember that learners' interests can change over time. For example, if a child learner is playing with a toy bus and a trainer wants to work on color identification, the trainer should not replace the bus with a stack of flash cards the child previously showed interest in.

Attention

A successful response is unlikely if a learner is not paying attention to an RBT's requests. As a result, it is crucial to make sure that the trainer has the learner's attention before initiating any action requiring a reaction.

Trainers should position themselves to have as many face-to-face interactions as possible. Getting close and at eye level helps the learner focus and understand what is expected.

For example, a child's attention can be caught by doing something unexpected or taking a turn with the desired toy.

Environment

As the learner dictates activities, the technician must have some control over the environment as well. This process allows for shared control, meaning if learners want to indulge in an activity, they must first go through the trainer.

Placing the desired item out of reach (but still keeping it visible) allows the learner to request it. Similarly, offering a small amount of an item increases the likelihood that the learner will request more in the future.

The learner can function without becoming overwhelmed if the environment is organized and the amount of visual, auditory or sensory stimuli are adjusted. A trainer, for example, arranges the play area so toys are stored in clear containers and separated by category.

To gain access to toys, the child learner must seek assistance from the trainer. As only one bucket is opened at a time, the child is not overstimulated by a toy-filled floor and thus the involvement in a specific toy is increased.

Time Delay

The trainer should wait for the learner's reaction after initiating or requesting something. This break gives the learner a chance to begin and allows time to process.

The instructor can encourage the learner to reply by employing nonverbal clues, like an expectant gaze, a questioning expression or body language. The trainer can provide further prompts or model the appropriate reaction if nonverbal clues are insufficient to get students to respond on their own.

Contingent Reinforcement

Reinforcement should be given contingent upon the learner exhibiting the desired behavior. For example, the trainer grants the learner's request and then offers chips.

The trainer should deny the request if the learner did not ask for chips but instead started complaining. Any tries and guesses should also be strengthened. The trainer should give the learner a chip to reward good behavior if the learner points and says "Chip" rather than "Chips."

Repetitive Reinforcement

Learners require multiple chances to practice a newly acquired skill. When first learning a skill, repetition may be back to back, but it is later scattered throughout the day to promote independence.

External conditions also contribute to the formation of opportunities for repetition. Offering small amounts ensures the learner repeats the action and requests more. Turns can also be used to interrupt play and allow for repetition.

Varying Difficulty Levels

Retaining motivation is a final point to consider while optimizing learning possibilities in the natural environment. The learners will remain interested if you follow their lead, and you can motivate them by altering the difficulty or giving them easier tasks.

For example, learners may be more inclined to keep going if they succeed and are challenged again.

Also, when challenging activities are combined with simple ones, frustration is kept to a minimum, reinforcement chances are increased and relationships succeed.

Task Analysis and Chaining Procedures

A task analysis is a behavior intervention that links a series of behaviors to form a more complex behavior chain. It can teach clients how to perform tasks, such as eating in the cafeteria, completing and turning in work, etc.

Task analysis is also helpful in desensitization programs, such as teaching learners to tolerate haircuts, brush teeth and deal with buzzers or loud environments.

Remember, what we consider simple may be complex for those on the spectrum. So, the intervention chain must be built before the intervention. The clients' skill set should also be considered when selecting appropriate interventions. All the steps must be specified.

An example of task analysis is given below.

How to Put on a Jacket

1. Pick up the jacket by grabbing its collar (the inside should be facing you).
2. Place your right arm through the right sleeve opening.
3. Extend your arm until you can see your hand at the other end.
4. Push your shoulders forward and extend your left arm behind yourself.
5. Put your left arm through the left sleeve opening.
6. Extend your arm until you can see your hand at the other end.
7. Pull the front of the jacket together.
8. Zip up the jacket.

The task analysis can be validated in three ways:

- Observing a competent person carry out the sequence of actions
- Consulting an expert or someone highly knowledgeable about the tasks to be taught
- Executing the entire series on your own

Task analysis involves the following behavior chains:

Forward Chaining

Forward chaining occurs when the first step—prompted or unprompted—is reinforced after the client completes and fully integrates the first step. The client usually does not move to the second step until the first step has been mastered.

For example, when dealing with children, forward chaining works for putting on shirts, making sandwiches, brushing teeth and a variety of other personal tasks.

Backward Chaining

Backward chaining begins with assistance with all steps except the last. When the previous step is done correctly, it is reinforced.

At each session, the reinforcement is backed through the chain, reinforcing the end of the sequence of known steps.

Backward chaining teaches the sequence, starting with the last step. Again, the previous step is not taught until the final step is understood.

Backward Chaining with a Leap Ahead

The procedure is similar to backward chaining, but not all task analysis steps are explicitly taught. Steps can be skipped. The leap ahead procedure reduces the training time required to learn the chain.

Total Task Chaining

Total task chaining consists of completing the entire sequence and receiving reinforcement at the end of the task chain. It is appropriate when the learner possesses the necessary skills to complete the tasks in the chain and does not require trials to criteria based on previously learned knowledge.

Whatever strategy is chosen, data must be collected to document the successful completion of the entire routine and progress on individual steps. Data collection is required to determine how an individual progresses through the task analysis steps and what strategies are used.

Discrimination Training

Discrimination refers to a learner's ability to understand the differences between two or more things.

During training, we frequently refer to various language operands, such as tact, intraverbal, etc. When we talk about receptive language, we mean the client's ability to take in and comprehend words.

Are the clients able to follow simple instructions? Are they aware the word *book* refers to the object we are reading? These are the fundamental building blocks of language development. Discrimination training is an essential component of that growth.

There are several types of discrimination training, including:

<u>Simultaneous Discrimination</u>

Simultaneous discrimination makes learners distinguish between two or more stimuli at the same time. It can be conducted in the following ways:

1. **Mass Trials** – This is a procedure in which you repeatedly present trials of the same simple discrimination. For example, you could consider placing a toy cat on the table (with no other toys present) and telling the learner to touch the cat. The learner is expected to respond by touching the cat. The trial would then be repeated several times in a row, with correct responses reinforced.
2. **Mass Trial with a Distractor** – This is a mass trial with one other stimulus. For example, place a toy dog and a toy cat on the table and present trials in which you ask the learner to touch the dog while changing the toys' positions frequently.
3. **Random Rotation** – This involves putting two or more stimuli and alternating between asking for each at random. For example, place a larger and a smaller cup on the table and ask, "Which is larger?" This is the most challenging level of discrimination.

Successive Discrimination

Successive discrimination happens when we do one thing in the presence of one stimulus and then do something else later in the presence of another stimulus.

For example, if you say, "Tell me about something that flies," the subsequent trial will be, "Tell me about something that swims."

Chapter 6: Transfer Control and Maintenance Procedures

Stimulus Control Procedures

Any difference observed in responding in the presence of different stimuli is called stimulus control. Behaviors in our everyday life involve stimulus control in some way.

The simplest way to explain stimulus control would be by considering a driver putting his foot on the brake pedal to respond to a red light.

However, when the same driver removes his foot from the accelerator when a green light is visible, the driver's response is under stimulus control of the light's color.

The process of analyzing stimulus control is central to the understanding of normal and abnormal behavior. These procedures are used to generate behavioral baselines for studying the effects of drugs and other physical implications.

Stimulus control procedures are descriptive solutions to changing how behavior is triggered. This can be done by the presence or absence of a stimulus.

Stimulus control is responsible for either prompting or inhibiting behavior. For example, a student is very talkative with her friends but quiet in class. Therefore, the student's social environment is responsible for exerting stimulus control over talking.

Transfer of Stimulus Control

Techniques that involve prompts being discontinued after the target behavior has started being displayed in the presence of SD are known as stimulus control transfer procedures.

These procedures successfully connect a stimulus with action and add another stimulus that leads to the same action. In other words, the transfer of stimulus control involves changing the cue. For instance, if the initial cue is a spoken command, this might be changed to a hand signal.

Simply put, the new stimulus is presented first, followed by the current one. When the subject completes the action, the connection is reinforced by a reward. The RBT continues doing this while reducing the current stimulus.

Initially, what needs to be kept in mind is that the new stimulus is apparent. With time, however, it can be reduced and made more subtle.

For example, a child is conditioned by her mother to come to the dinner table when called. The child, however, only obeys the command when the mother calls and not when the father calls.

So, the mother and the father work together, calling the child while the mother steps back. Eventually, the mother stops stepping back and the child begins coming to the dinner table, obeying the commands of both parents equally.

The example shows that the subject needs to be fully under stimulus control to not be confused. If new cues lead to reduced performance when the original cue is being used, the transfer of control should be delayed to a future date.

Prompt and Prompt-Fading Procedures

Sometimes the client does not produce correct responses to instructions. In other words, the client does not independently make the right responses to instructions or commands. This can also happen while learning new skills. In such instances, prompting may be required.

The addition of cues with instruction that can increase the likelihood of the student being able to produce correct responses is known as prompting. When a client has access to reinforcement for responding correctly, the possibility of the behavior occurring more often increases.

Depending on the level of intrusiveness, there are several types of prompts. The prompt selection should be based on what the student requires to be successful.

For teaching new skills, most to least prompting is considered beneficial. This involves the most intrusive level of prompt required for student success.

However, when learned or mastered skills are to be reviewed, least to most prompting can be used.

The vital thing to keep in mind is that all prompts should be reduced as soon as they are no longer required. This is important because prompt dependency can occur if the student has learned to give the correct response only in the presence of a prompt.

Types of Prompts

Prompting procedures involve removing and providing prompts so the learner can independently perform a particular behavior. They include the following:

Gestural Prompts

As the name suggests, the gestural prompt involves gestures or any action the subject can observe. This can include nodding, pointing and reaching out—all of which can give information about the correct response.

- **Full Physical Prompts**

Full physical prompts involve physically guiding the subject's hands to help complete the task. They are considered the most intrusive prompt and are also known as hand-over-hand assistance.

- **Partial Physical Prompts**

When using partial physical prompts, the instructor guides the subject through part of the assigned activity. This is a less intrusive method than a full physical prompt.

- **Verbal Prompts**

Verbal prompts involve showing the subject a visible picture or cue, such as a video, drawing, flash card, etc.

- **Positional Prompts**

In this procedure, the correct response is placed closest to the learner to help provide information.

Prompt Fading

The reduction or removal of prompts paired with instruction is known as prompt fading. It allows the learner to perform independently.

Prompt fading also prevents the learner from getting dependent on the prompt and involves removing the prompt quickly.

Prompt fading includes three main elements:

- **Physical**

A complete physical prompt is faded to a partial physical prompt. It involves decreasing the level of intrusiveness, which is done by following the prompt hierarchy using most to least prompting.

- **Time Delay**

Time delay involves increasing the use of prompts by gradually increasing the length of time between the instruction and delivery time.

- **Proximity**

Proximity involves introducing a systematic change in the spatial positions of the learner.

Generalization and Maintenance Procedures

Generalization

When behavior is performed outside the learning environment, generalization occurs. It takes place through various dimensions without learning and can happen across settings, time and people.

In generalization, an individual will apply something learned in a specific situation to similar situations marked by progress toward the therapy goal. This is also known as carryover.

Carryover applies to the situation when a client's progress is seen outside the therapy setting, such as the home, school, parks, etc. However, it can also include multiple people, such as parents, caregivers, teachers, etc.

Furthermore, carryover is not an automatic procedure and requires constant work, which ensures the change in behavior becomes meaningful. The process involves practicing skills to ensure the person who uses these skills can utilize them when required in any given situation or environment.

Generalization Methods

There are several generalization methods.

Teaching Multiple Examples

Teaching multiple examples is one of the most reliable ways of generalization and can be applied across several settings and multiple people.

Teaching Across Multiple People

If a client has several different teachers, teaching across multiple people will be most efficient. When different people teach the client, their instruction will allow the child to perform an action with a variety of people.

Teaching with Multiple Instructions

For a client with autism, learning and understanding different instructions can be a bit difficult. So, it is advised to start by giving one instruction, then giving another, which is constantly reinforced.

Choosing Functional Behavior

Choosing functional behavior involves teaching the client behaviors that are useful in everyday life. This allows the client to independently get reinforcement from the environment—a result of behavioral change.

Maintenance

The continued performance of a skill after all teaching has stopped is known as maintenance. In other words, maintenance occurs if a client can perform a specific behavior after the teaching process for that particular behavior has stopped.

Maintenance can also be described as the client's ability to demonstrate previously acquired skills over time. It is measured by reviewing the fact that reinforcement has reduced below the level at which the skill was initially taught.

The learner needs to be able to continue performing the behaviors taught even after the teaching is over. To ensure that, it is crucial to design a teaching program that involves the learner being taught not just simple skills, but skills that could be used in daily life.

For example, teaching certain words to every client might be unnecessary. This is because some words might be helpful for one client but useless for another.

Shaping Procedures

In ABA, *shaping* can be defined as the reinforcement of successive approximations of the desired behavior. In other words, the process involves reinforcing the client whenever approximations of the desired behavior are demonstrated.

However, the client is not reinforced if approximations of the desired behavior are not performed.

Another way of defining shaping is a process or technique in which a behavioral skill is taught to a client by providing reinforcement whenever the desired behavior is performed. It helps teach new skills to the learner, as it is an aspect of behavior analysis.

Clearly defining the behavioral objective is necessary for shaping to be effective and successful. RBTs must also know precisely when to reinforce the client and when to withhold reinforcement.

RBTs must also use their clients' knowledge and behaviors and consider the skill they wish to teach the clients before using shaping.

<u>**The Initial Process**</u>

In the initial process, before the actual procedure begins, the RBT must perform a few steps to ensure the best possible outcome. These steps include the following:

1. **Choose the Target Behavior** – The RBT needs to know what behavior is required to be achieved. This makes it easier for the client to understand exactly how things proceed because clarity is needed.
2. **Determine the Student's Present Performance Level** – During the procedure, the RBT must know what the client is and is not currently doing. This will help determine the exact behavior required to be performed.
3. **List the Steps Needed to Achieve the Target Behavior** – Before beginning to teach, the RBT must list all the steps to the target behavior. This makes the process move forward systematically.
4. **Teach the Client the First Step** – When the prescribed approximation of the target behavior has been exhibited, the RBT can reinforce the client.
5. **Make the Behavior Extinct** – If the client exhibits the reinforced behavior reliably, the behavior must be put on extinction and only closer approximations to the target behavior should be reinforced. This strategy should continue until the target behavior is not achieved.

How to Use Shaping

The shaping process begins with a task analysis. In this analysis, the desired behavior is broken down into smaller steps that are easier to manage. The aim is to move the client closer to the desired behavior.

For example, if playing independently for 10 minutes is the desired behavior (with two or fewer prompts), a task analysis will help break the target behavior into approximations as follows:

1. Playing for two minutes with a maximum of two prompts
2. Playing for four minutes with a maximum of two prompts
3. Playing for six minutes with a maximum of two prompts
4. Plying for eight minutes with a maximum of two prompts
5. Playing for 10 minutes with a maximum of two prompts

After clearly identifying the approximations of the desired behavior, the reinforcement that needs to be used should be selected. Also, everyone working with the client should know the target behavior and how to reinforce it.

Lastly, the team involved should collect and review the data regarding the procedure. The program must continue until the client does not start independently demonstrating the desired behavior.

An example describing the use of this procedure is a child not sitting quietly in class for a lecture. The desired behavior for the child is to remain seated for 20 minutes. Considering the shaping method, the child will be observed and reinforced for close approximations of the desired behavior.

The child will be reinforced for the first time for being seated for two minutes straight. The second time the child will be reinforced for being seated for five minutes. This will continue until the child remains seated for 20 minutes, which is the target behavior.

Token Economy Procedures

A token economy involves the delivery of a tangible conditioned reinforcer by using a contingency-based procedure developed to aid in the reduction of maladaptive behaviors.

In this procedure, the frequency of a target behavior is reinforced. Tokens or symbols are provided to the client when the target behavior is performed. The client can then exchange these same tokens for other kinds of reinforcement, such as treats or snacks.

A token economy is a reinforcement strategy that involves generalized reinforcers and backup reinforcers:

- **Generalized Reinforcers** – These are rewards or tokens the RBT gives every time the target behavior is exhibited. These generalized reinforcers can be collected by the client and be exchanged with backup reinforcers.
- **Backup Reinforcers** – These are rewards the client gets by exchanging the collected token, such as candy, treats or snacks.

Once clients are aware that collecting rewards will give them access to another kind of reward, the clients might repeat the behavior. Eventually, the clients might learn to exhibit the behavior independently, even without being reinforced.

For example, a target behavior provided by the RBT is asking for help rather than screaming out loud. Every time the client performs the desired behavior, given the stimulus, "Do you have a question?" the RBT will reinforce the client by providing a token.

When the client successfully collects five to 10 tokens, they can be exchanged for another form of reinforcement, such as a treat or a snack.

Section 4: Behavior Reduction

Chapter 7: The Function of Behavior

What Is Behavior?

In ABA, anything a person says or does is referred to as behavior. In other words, behavior means observable actions. This also includes things that can be seen and that cannot be seen. In ABA, things that can be seen are overt behavior, while things that cannot be seen are called covert behavior. Feelings and emotions are covert behaviors.

Covert behaviors explain a feeling, such as happiness or sadness. Even though these feelings are valid, they are often characterized by the BCBA as overt feelings that people can see to present a better understanding of the behavior.

Measurable Behavior

In ABA, behavior is supposed to be explained in a way that makes it measurable. This makes data analysis easy, and the RBT can then help change the behavior without much effort.

Now, how does covert behavior become measurable? Being hungry is a behavior. However, this behavior cannot be measured. But when a hungry person eats something in front of the RBT, the action can be observed and measured. So, the behavior of hunger will be measured by noting the behavioral aspects visible to the RBT.

Sometimes behavior cannot be seen if it is covert. So, in these situations, the RBT must look for signs of covert behavior. For example, sadness itself cannot be measured if a client is sad. However, the number of times the client cries due to sadness or the kind of tone the client uses when speaking can be measured.

The critical thing to understand is that even though the client's feelings or thoughts are not being measured, the actions related to those feelings or thoughts are.

While the observation is not direct, the behavior measured is not inaccurate as the overt behavior is generated from the covert behavior. So, a measurement or observation of the result of the covert behavior is the measurement of the covert behavior itself.

Effecting change in a client's behavior is not possible without measurement, which is why it is essential that even when the client is feeling something, the RBT must look for other signs to identify what is happening inside the individual.

This observation helps when the client is not communicating with the RBT properly. RBTs can only help their clients if they know what is going on with an individual or what exactly a person is feeling.

Functions of Behavior

In ABA, RBTs use functions of behavior to identify why a behavior occurs. These are also used to prevent behavior and choose a replacement for certain behavior.

Functions of behavior can also be used for creating behavior plans. There are four functions of behavior in ABA therapy:

Sensory Stimulation

Sensory stimulation includes movements and actions that feel good to the individual. These actions can be a result of seeking satisfaction or coping with a particular situation.

An example of sensory stimulation is twirling the hair after being seated for an extended time. These actions occur when an individual is seeking sensory input. So, if the action being performed provides the necessary sensory input the individual seeks, the action will continue.

Escape

Escapist behavior can be described as an individual trying to escape a situation that does not feel comfortable or desirable. As a result, the individual will act in a way that helps the person escape the task.

A simple example is a child running away after being told to brush his teeth. The child will show escapist behavior if the process of brushing his teeth is not desirable or satisfying for him.

However, an escape does not need to be a physical retaliation toward the assigned task. Instead, it can also be presented as a signal that confirms the individuals do not want to do what is asked of them. These signals do not have to be extreme and are often enough to be measured and observed.

Access to Attention

Access-to-attention behaviors occur when the client tries to get another person's attention. These behaviors are usually more prominent than others and stand out, fulfilling their purpose.

An example is a child screaming to gain a person's attention. This behavior is identified by noticing the intensity with which a behavior is performed. Similarly, another example is an adult waving her hands above her head.

Access to Tangibles

Access-to-tangibles behavior occurs when an individual wants access to something. It can be extreme and happens only when the individual actually wants something. In such a situation, the individual tries hard to get what he wants through his behavior.

An example is a boy pinching his brother when his toy is taken away from him. The behavior continues if it gets the individual the desired article. In this situation, if pinching gets the boy his toy back, he will use that strategy until he is asked not to.

The Function of Behavior

RBTs need to be able to identify functions of behavior to prevent problematic behavior. This is also important for ensuring consistency across all environments.

To identify a behavior, RBTs first note down the events that occur before and after the behavior occurs, identify the function and teach the client a replacement for the negative behavior.

Identifying the functions of behavior helps RBTs identify problematic behaviors, decrease them and increase appropriate and targeted behaviors.

Replacement Behaviors

While most people think a replacement behavior is a long-term, permanent behavior required for the client to learn new skills, it is the opposite.

A replacement behavior is a temporary, short-term replacement for another behavior. It is considered when the original behavior is inappropriate, causes clients stress or is unhealthy for them.

Replacing a behavior with another behavior helps clients learn new skills and cope with difficulties. As a result, clients can meet their needs while learning the skills to engage using the desired behavior.

The vital thing to remember is that the replacement behavior should be faster and easier than the original behavior of concern. This is important as it is the only way the client will try to implement the replacement behavior.

Also, the replacement behavior must be socially acceptable and a healthy alternative for the client.

If the replacement behavior is more complex and time-consuming than the actual behavior of concern, the client will likely continue with the original behavior.

An example of a replacement behavior is teaching a child to ask to be heard rather than interrupting another person's conversation by screaming or shouting. Both screaming and politely requesting will allow the client to fulfill his needs. However, screaming will not be socially acceptable or healthy for the client.

How to Choose a Replacement Behavior

Specific things need to be kept in mind when choosing replacement behaviors for the client.

First, the RBT needs to understand why a client might be engaging in the targeted behavior. A functional behavior assessment should be used to identify these concerns.

The main goal while finding a replacement behavior should be for clients to meet the exact purpose they are looking for. If the replacement behavior does not fulfill a client's needs, it will be of no use.

Keeping these things in mind makes it easy for RBTs to search for a replacement behavior. Eventually, improvement can be observed. Note that this kind of behavior is meant to be temporary.

Regardless of how efficient the replacement behavior is for the client, the main goal is to eradicate the inappropriate behavior and replace it with an appropriate behavior.

Transition Strategies

Transition strategies can be beneficial because they can help clients learn new skills quickly so they move forward efficiently with their learning process.

Clients with autism have difficulty transitioning from one task to another. This is why using different transitioning methods can help them effectively transition between tasks and learn how to cope or deal with anxiety and fear related to change.

Even though a change in environment is essential for children with ASD, some children find it challenging to cope with new environments and need sameness and predictability. However, their ability to learn and adapt can be affected if this learning environment is encouraged.

Types of Transition Strategies

The client must be the primary concern when choosing a transition strategy. The way these strategies are used also depends on the client.

Warning clients of the time limit ending will only cause them to be anxious, and completing the task will become even more difficult. This is why there are specific ways of dealing with clients in ABA when choosing transition strategies, including:

Visual Timer

Visual timers help clients understand how much time is left to complete the task. Timers go red when the time is almost up. This indication helps clients switch to the other task as the signal reminds them of their next step.

When the red indicator on the timer has dimmed, the clients will know it is time to transition.

Using Photos Icons or Words

Research has shown that visual objects can increase the probability of following a demanded behavior and decrease challenging behavior while transitioning into another task.

In this method, RBTs might use a photo, icon or word as a cue for the task they wish a client to transition to. Visually seeing a representation of the next task makes it easy for the client to transition.

However, the process can also be done through words. A simple word representing the demanded task can help the client understand when the transition needs to occur.

- **Reduction of Problem Behavior with Functional Communication**

The primary aim of functional communication is to make implementing replacement behavior easier and more effective. The replacement is done using more common forms of communication. However, several steps need to be considered to implement the replacement behavior fully.

An example is teaching the client that snatching or grabbing things from other people's hands is not the right way to ask for something. Instead, communicating with the other person by simply pointing at the object is a better, more appropriate behavior.

Clients are taught words and actions that can help them achieve their target and perform appropriate behavior at the same time.

Coping Strategies

Coping strategies help clients remain calm when problem behaviors occur. Instead of expressing themselves through inappropriate behaviors, RBTs help clients use alternative ways to calm down before moving forward. This could include exercises like silent counting, deep breathing and distraction.

Behavior Reduction Plan

A behavior reduction plan is created when ABA professionals deal with behavior they wish to reduce. It is the last step in the FBA process. After determining the function of the client's behavior, ABA professionals create a behavior reduction plan.

Determining the function of the behavior and creating a behavior plan go hand in hand; neither is complete without the other. The ABA professional needs to understand why a behavior occurs and decide what to do about that particular behavior. For that reason, a written behavior reduction plan has to be created.

The severity of the client's behavior determines who can create and write a behavior reduction plan. In some cases, even parents and teachers can create a behavior reduction plan. However, an ABA professional at the BCBA or BCaA level can always write a behavior reduction plan if needed.

Components of a Behavior Reduction Plan

Behavior reduction plans are usually used in schools, homes and community settings. They are essential to prevent and reduce problematic behavior. Implementing new ways to cope with inappropriate behavior can also be done with the help of a behavior reduction plan.

There are several components of a behavior reduction plan, including:

Identifying Information

The identifying information is where the basics of ABA sessions with a client are mentioned. It includes the intervention plan, the client's information, the stakeholders and the setting in which the goal is to be implemented.

Describing the Behavior

The behavior to be reduced must be mentioned clearly in the plan with a specific description.

Replacement Behaviors

The plan needs to include the replacement behaviors to be implemented in place of the behavior to be reduced. The replacement behaviors need to be socially acceptable and easier to perform than the target behavior.

Preventive Strategies

The plan should clearly mention ways to prevent the targeted undesirable behavior from occurring. This could include information like changing the environment or eliminating triggers.

Consequence Strategies

Consequential strategies help ABA professionals create a plan for what will follow in case of appropriate or inappropriate behavior.

For example, what should be the consequence if a child bangs items into tables, floors or walls to gain attention? And how should the RBT react if the child does not shout and waits for his turn to speak?

The consequence of such behavior should be mentioned in the plan. For instance, the plan could mention that inappropriate behavior will result in the loss of privileges for the child, while appropriate behavior might lead to the opposite.

Data Collection Procedures

While it is essential to mention the target behavior in the written plan, it is also important to mention it in a way that makes it observable and measurable.

If the person writing the plan wishes to make changes to the plan, the changes must be based on progress as indicated by the recorded data.

The Duration of the Plan

The duration of a plan mentions the amount of time in which the particular plan will be carried out.

The behavior reduction plan for a typical school setting should be one year. However, the duration also depends on the data collected about the client's behavior.

Chapter 8: Reinforcement Extinction and Emergency Procedures

Differential Reinforcement

There are many ways RBTs can try to change a problematic behavior, and differential reinforcement is one of them. In this kind of reinforcement, the learner receives reinforcement only for a specific behavior class and reinforcement for all the other behaviors is withheld.

For example, if the client's target behavior is to wash her hands, reinforcement will be possible only if the washing of hands occurs. Any other behavior will not be rewarded, even if it is appropriate.

The theory revolves around differential reinforcement: people tend to repeat behaviors that are reinforced, not behaviors that are not. There are two components of differential reinforcement:

1. Reinforcement for appropriate behavior
2. Withholding reinforcement for inappropriate behavior

Differential reinforcement can be considered the opposite of traditional discipline. The simplest way to describe this would be to encourage someone's positive behavior rather than discourage negative behavior.

For example, if someone's behavior is inappropriate, there will not be a punishment for that behavior. However, there would be a reward or reinforcement for the appropriate behavior. In this way, the person will remember the reinforcement rather than the punishment and the reinforced behavior will likely be repeated.

When someone is not reinforced for inappropriate behavior, this is called withholding the reinforcement. It means ignoring the inappropriate behavior. However, there are specific ways to ignore such behavior. RBTs will usually make eye contact, remain silent or move away when inappropriate behavior occurs.

The chances of success with differential reinforcement will increase only when the client is reinforced immediately after performing the desired behavior. This quick response to the behavior will help the client understand the importance of the appropriate behavior. Since this behavior will result in positive reinforcement, the client will likely perform it again.

Types of Differential Reinforcement

There are four types of differential reinforcement:

Differential Reinforcement of Incompatible Behavior (DRI)

There are some behaviors that, despite being alternative behaviors, are not compatible with the problem behavior. The DRI procedure entails that only those behaviors that cannot simultaneously occur with the problem behavior must be reinforced.

An example of the DRI procedure is a child screaming to get something done. As a result, the RBT will consider the DRI procedure. Calmly asking for a required article will be chosen as the incompatible behavior, as it cannot occur at the same time as screaming for something.

So, the RBT will reinforce the child for calmly requesting things, and reinforcement will be withheld whenever the child screams for things.

Differential Reinforcement of Alternative Behavior (DRA)

In this procedure, certain behaviors are reinforced, serving as an alternative to the problem behavior. However, these behaviors are not necessarily incompatible with the problem behavior. The problem behavior and the alternative can sometimes co-occur, but reinforcement will occur only for the socially appropriate behavior.

For example, a little girl is told to raise her hand every time she wishes to ask a question in class. However, she instead chooses to shout to be heard. So, she will be reinforced only when she raises her hand.

Differential Reinforcement of Other Behavior (DRO)

In this procedure, a client is reinforced if the problem behavior has not occurred for a predetermined time. RBTs will usually set timers for the client; if the problem behavior does not happen during that time, the client is reinforced. However, the timer is reset if the client continues with the problem behavior.

For instance, a child is banging the table repeatedly while performing an independent task. The RBT will let the child know that a timer is being set, and the child will be asked to follow instructions by remaining calm and not banging his fists against the table.

If the timer is set for three minutes, the child must remain calm for that time. There should be an absence of the problem behavior during that time.

Differential Reinforcement of Low Rates (DRL)

This procedure is not used for problem behaviors but rather behaviors that occur too often. If a client is indulging in repetitive behaviors and these behaviors are becoming unhealthy, the RBT will consider DRL.

In this procedure, the client will be reinforced if the behavior does not occur within the predetermined amount of time and is below the predetermined criteria.

For example, a child begins greeting his peers in class, which is appropriate behavior. However, it is problematic if he starts doing this 10 times during a class.

The child will then be reinforced if the behavior does not occur during the predetermined time or if the quantity of behavioral repetitions begins to lower.

Extinction Procedures in ABA

In ABA, extinction is withholding or discontinuing the reinforcement for the problem behavior to decrease the occurrences of negative behaviors.

Extinction procedures usually take three different forms, depending on the functions of behavior, including:

Extinction of Behaviors Maintained by Positive Reinforcement

In this procedure, inappropriate behaviors will not be reinforced in any way. Instead, they will be ignored to reduce the probability of their reoccurrence.

An example is a child dropping toys to catch her parent's attention. If the parent responds to the child by giving her attention or picking up the toy, the child's needs will be fulfilled. As a result, the child will continue with the behavior.

So, to make this behavior extinct, the parent ignores the child or gently chides her for her actions.

Extinction of Behavior Maintained by Negative Reinforcement

Another form of the extinction of behavior includes behaviors maintained by negative reinforcement. It is also referred to as escape extinction.

To explain this procedure, consider the example of a boy throwing tantrums for not wanting to complete the assigned work. In such a situation, if the child's teacher punishes him, the child's needs will be fulfilled as the work will not be done and the boy will get a chance to avoid work.

To reduce this kind of problematic behavior, the child must be ignored and allowed to throw tantrums regardless of how long he takes to quiet down. Meanwhile, the teacher must continue encouraging the child to complete his work.

In such situations, the screaming and shouting might be aggravated initially, but the problematic behavior will decrease with time.

Extinction of Behaviors Maintained by Automatic Reinforcement

This procedure is commonly referred to as sensory extinction. Sensory stimulation that attracts a problematic behavior should be removed in this procedure. If the client does not get the sensory stimulation from the behavior, the behavior will not continue.

For example, a child loves to switch on fans. In such a situation, if the fan is disabled, the child will no longer get the sensory stimulation the fan was previously providing. So, there would be a higher chance of the behavior not taking place in the future.

The Aftermath of Extinction Procedures

Negative behavior is likely to increase after the implementation of the extinction procedure. This increase in negative behavior is known as an extinction burst. However, RBTs must continue with the procedure regarding the client's behavior.

There will be an increase in the problematic behavior, but this will decrease to an appropriate level. Sometimes problematic behavior might not occur suddenly after the extinction procedures but might come back after a long period when the child has not performed any challenging behaviors. This is called spontaneous recovery.

RBTs need to be prepared for this possibility. All the forms of extinction mentioned above can decrease the probability of inappropriate behavior.

Preventive Intervention

Understanding the reason for the occurrence of behavior is a better way of decreasing it rather than designing interventions based on what behavior may look like.

When behavior reduction plans are absent, RBTs can use other techniques to deal with aggressive behavior. The critical thing to note here is that these techniques do not eliminate problematic behavior a client might display, but they can help end aggressive episodes safely.

Neutral Redirection

This procedure involves redirection from one behavior to another. In this procedure, the client's inappropriate behavior will be observed and the individual will be guided to perform a functionally appropriate behavior instead.

For instance, when using the neutral redirection procedure, a child's inappropriate behavior must not be paid attention to, as it will increase the probability of the behavior continuing.

If a child keeps hitting others when told to perform a specific task, the inappropriate behavior must not be provided any attention. Instead, quietly moving away, ignoring the child and repeating the demanded task will be sufficient neutral redirection.

RBTs can also redirect clients by suggesting an alternative behavior for the inappropriate behavior. For example, hitting someone to get their attention could be replaced with slowly tapping a person on the shoulder.

Attention and Praise

In this kind of procedure, inappropriate behavior will not be given any attention. Instead, the appropriate behavior will be praised.

Sometimes if an RBT finds a client is showing appropriate behavior, the client will receive praise for it, increasing the chances of the behavior occurring more often.

Other than that, clients can also be given a list of tasks and a choice to choose the task they wish to complete. This, too, will help reduce problematic behavior.

Making the learning environment comfortable and friendly will also help the client choose appropriate behavior more often.

Preventative Measures

Specific strategies can be considered in addition to preventive intervention. However, they cannot replace the need for behavior reduction plans. Instead, they provide ABA professionals with ways of dealing with aggressive behavior.

Following are some strategies that can help with the reduction of problematic behavior.

Visual Stimulation

If children are provided with a visual schedule, including a list of activities they need to complete, it will become easier for them to choose which tasks they need to perform first and last.

The schedule will give the children freedom of choice and decrease problematic behavior in the future.

Rewards

When a person is rewarded for appropriate behavior, the chances of that behavior occurring again begin to increase. So, rather than focusing on what the client is doing wrong, the RBT can focus on the things the client is doing right and reinforce them.

Motivation and Reinforcement

Certain things motivate a client. Once the RBT has identified these things, they can be used as rewards for appropriate behavior.

Rewarding clients with something they like might increase the chances of proper behavior occurring more often. For example, if an RBT has determined a client likes to watch documentaries, he could reward the client with documentaries once the individual completes an appropriate behavior.

However, rewarding a client too often can lead to dependency and decrease independence of action. So, RBTs should take a measured approach when using this strategy.

Protecting Yourself

When working with a client who is showing aggressive behavior, it is essential for RBTs to protect themselves.

Wearing clothing that covers body areas likely to be targeted during the display of aggression is extremely important. It is also important to cover or contain the hair.

RBTs must remain mindful of when the client may act aggressively and act accordingly.

Section 5: Documentation and Reporting

Chapter 9: Communication, Supervision and Clinical Directions

RBTs are supervised by a BCBA RBT supervisor. RBTs make ABA therapy more accessible to people with autism and other behavioral disorders.

To start with the basics, to become a BCBA, you must have a master's degree. However, only a high school diploma is required to acquire an RBT certificate.

Aside from that, a BCBA goes through an extensive course of study and a 90-minute exam to gain certification, which is why only a board-certified behavior analyst (BCBA) can supervise them.

RBT Supervision Under BCBA

According to the BCBA, anyone acquiring ABA training must meet stringent requirements to achieve certification. One of these requirements includes being supervised by the BCBA.

Usually, a candidate's supervised experience can be accumulated within the employment setting.

Supervision is essential for several reasons. First, being supervised by a professional helps increase your confidence about the work you will do for your future clients. Secondly, a supervisor may help you realize and resolve problem areas in your skills.

It is essential to understand that while RBTs require supervision by a BCBA, the supervision is not counted unless the RBT has been supervised for a certain number of hours in a month.

Even though the quality of the supervision is initially necessary, the quantity of supervision is actually required to qualify as an RBT.

Supervision can be conducted by a qualified RBT supervisor and is a necessary part of the supervision requirements for an RBT. It helps an RBT maintain professional and ethical standards and facilitates the delivery of high-quality services.

RBT supervisors are responsible for the work performed by RBTs, which is why they must provide ongoing supervision. This is also why RBTs must meet requirements at every organization where RBT service is provided.

How Is an RBT Supervised?

The RBT task list demonstrates a list of activities the RBT needs to perform. During supervision, the BCBA has the discretion to decide whether or not the RBT has competently performed these activities.

The amount of supervision required is 5%. So, if an RBT works 100 hours a month, he or she must be supervised for at least five hours a month.

RBT supervision consists of developing performance expectations and reviewing written material, for example, data sheets, daily progress notes, etc. For an RBT, it is imperative to model technical, professional and ethical behavior with clients.

Observing behavioral skills and delivering performance feedback is also necessary for supervisors.

The Structure

RBT supervision has some specific requirements, and the structure of supervision depends upon that. At least two real-time face-to-face meetings are required.

The supervisor should be able to observe the RBT providing services at least once during the monthly meetings. This is required for an in-person, on-site observation of the RBT.

Even though an evaluation of a working RBT is necessary for supervision, it can be done through webcams and other online platforms instead of the supervisor being physically present.

Aside from that, at least one-on-one supervision is required—where only the RBT and the BCBA supervisor are present. However, other meetings can be held in groups where other RBTs with similar experiences participate.

Supervisors are responsible for the services RBTs provide. As a result, they must hold a BCBA certification or should be licensed in another behavioral health profession.

In organizations with many RBTs and RBT supervisors, one person is designated to serve as the RBT requirements coordinator.

The RBT requirements coordinator is responsible for ensuring the organization meets every supervision requirement. The coordinator can also serve as an RBT supervisor.

Communication and Supervision

Effective communication is essential during supervision. The RBT and the supervisor need to ensure their communication skills are both receptive and expressive to discuss issues and problem areas promptly and without rancor.

An RBT must follow the supervisor's directions by taking in the information provided. Keeping these directions in mind during meetings and face-to-face communication is vital. Reviewing the information suggested by the supervisor can help RBTs become better at their job.

Both the RBT and the supervisor must have a mutual understanding of the situation being analyzed, so effective communication is vital. This is involved in receptive communication skills, where information provided by the supervisor is analyzed.

As far as expressive skills are concerned, this responsibility lies in the hands of the RBT. Providing supervisors with complete information about the client's progress and functioning is imperative. In contrast, when providing RBT services, any concerns about the client must be discussed with the supervisor. This also includes reporting any incidents that have occurred.

It is critical during supervision to use the correct ABA terminology to address matters. This helps supervisors ensure that RBT principles are being practiced effectively.

While the main concern is always the client, supervisors need to be told about caregivers as well. This includes family members, community helpers, etc.

Steps to Ensure Effective Communication During Supervision

RBT supervisors have limitations and boundaries regarding how much time they can give an RBT and when they can be available to talk.

Effective communication can be possible only if the RBT chooses an appropriate time to speak with the supervisor and gives the supervisor enough time to analyze the data. So, rushing a supervisor will not ensure effectiveness.

Even though supervisors should be contacted for appointments or meetings, some issues need immediate solutions and need to be discussed right away. It is the RBT's responsibility to know which kinds of issues need to be addressed immediately and which do not.

The RBT's behavior toward the supervisor determines whether or not the person should be given the responsibility of taking care of clients. An RBT must always behave professionally.

Another critical step in ensuring effective communication is accepting feedback and responding appropriately.

RBTs can express their opinions; however, it is also necessary to understand their role in complying with the supervisor's treatment plan.

Seeking Clinical Direction

The supervision of a particular client's case is referred to as clinical direction. According to practice guidelines given by the BCBA, several activities are involved in seeking clinical direction—mostly on the part of the professional behavior analyst or RBT. The guidelines demonstrate that multiple variables determine the appropriate intensity and other aspects of case supervision.

According to the guidelines, the general standard of care involves two hours of supervision for every 10 hours of direct treatment. The individual client's needs must be considered, as they are responsive to the amount of supervision for each case.

A client's ASD symptoms are reflected by the ratio of case supervision hours to direct treatment hours, meaning the supervision hours listed within the guidelines are just a general parameter. If the RBT determines a particular number of hours are required for case supervision, then these hours need to be authorized.

Authorized hours may need adjustment throughout the client's treatment. They do not substitute for hours of direct ABA treatment.

Chapter 10: Reporting and Compliance

Several factors need to be considered when offering RBT services to clients. These factors relate to the functioning of a client's behaviors.

Even though the antecedents and consequences of a client's behavior are the most common factors considered for a client's functioning, an RBT must also look at other factors that might be playing a role in the client's behavior.

Setting Events

Setting events appear in different ways. They can include illnesses, lack of sleep and changes in the client's mood, as well as changes in biological needs, such as hunger.

For example, the reaction of a sleepless little boy to his toy being taken away would differ from his reaction to the situation when he has had enough sleep. The boy is likely to throw a tantrum because of lack of sleep, and the situation could be used as an example to analyze the boy's behaviors.

It is possible that if the boy has had enough sleep, he might be willing to share his toy rather than cry about it.

Importance of Reporting Setting Behaviors

Other variables that can alter a client's behavior include illnesses. Medications can also affect behavior. Thus, it is the RBTs responsibility to be aware of these variables to offer effective services to clients.

Clients might behave a certain way due to these variables. While some of these variables might have the potential to be ignored, the RBT is responsible for determining the cause of the client's behavior through further observation and evaluation.

Setting Events

Setting events must be reported immediately, as these count as events leading up to certain behaviors. Once the setting event is confirmed, it becomes easier to understand the client's triggers.

However, it must be noted that even though a setting event leads to the main trigger, it is not the trigger itself. Actual triggers can take place days and even months before the actual behavior.

So, even though simple variables, like lack of sleep and hunger, can cause behavioral changes, an unstable home and work life can have the same effect on a client. This is why speaking to the client's family and friends can help RBTs understand behavior.

While some variables might be constant, like unstable home life, others occur occasionally. For example, if a client argues with someone, that can trigger a certain behavior. So, determining the actual setting event for a particular behavior is an essential responsibility of the RBT.

Communication

Once an RBT has determined a particular setting event is indeed present and altering the client's behavior, the RBT must initiate communication. It is often challenging to understand the trigger behind negative behavior. Determining a single trigger might not be enough.

Communication can help correct the setting event and make it possible to control the negative behavior in the future. This can start with either the client or the client's surroundings depending upon the determined setting event reported by the RBT.

Medication and Illnesses

Regarding medication and illnesses, reporting these variables is also crucial, as any setting event can be managed if it is analyzed in time.

For instance, a client suffering from a medical condition will require constant support and motivation. Once the variable causing the alteration of the client's behavior is reported, the RBT can begin using different ways to deal with the setting event.

Often the client's family is unaware of what is causing negative behavior, which is why an early analysis of any of these variables is necessary for effective results.

Generating Objective Session Notes

When working with clients, taking notes objectively and professionally is essential. Objective notes include factual observation and information used for and revealed by the client's evaluation.

On the other hand, personal notes include the RBT's thoughts about the session. Since these notes are added to the client's permanent record, RBTs must write them using professional language.

The session notes can include the setting of the client's environment and how it might have influenced the client's behavior throughout the session. While mentioning these variables in the notes, it is also crucial to have an objective approach.

For instance, if an RBT knows the client argued with a family member before the session, this must be mentioned in the session notes. This is an example of objective reasoning.

Objective notes help other RBTs who might work with the client understand the situation in depth. Thus, documenting the entire session is extremely important.

Consulting Third Parties

RBTs might collaborate with other professionals or supervisors. When this happens, the client's best interest must be kept in mind and clients should be informed about the collaboration. Since clients have a right to privacy, the client's consent must involve a third party in the therapy process.

Even though the BCBA is the supervising authority for RBTs, there are some other professionals or experts an RBT might consult, such as speech-language pathologists, physical therapists, special education teachers and many others.

The RBT may collaborate with these experts to make sure the client gets the best service possible and to ensure the effectiveness of the treatment.

ABC Data Documentation

The ABC data form is an assessment tool for analyzing a client's behavior. This tool evolves into a data implementation plan. A stands for *antecedent*, B for *behavior* and C for *consequences*.

The RBT is not directly responsible for collecting ABC data. Rather a trained person should be present to collect data when a particular behavior is displayed.

For ABC data collection, it is necessary to understand that simulating a behavior by creating a situation should be avoided. For example, if something close to the client is taken away and the client becomes upset, creating a situation where a client's favorite item is taken away should be avoided.

What Should Session Notes Include?

RBTs write session notes at the end of each session. During the session, the RBT can take notes regarding objective observation.

While RBTs are allowed to add their input, it is necessary to have the majority of the session notes written accurately and objectively. This provides a neutral report for the functioning of the client's behavior and makes it easier to understand the client's behavior and think of possible steps to take.

While writing session notes, the RBT must mention the client's name and the date and time the session is being conducted. In other words, all real-time information is to be mentioned in the session notes.

Other than that, the type of visit should also be mentioned, along with the length of the visit. This will help determine how many hours a week the RBT communicates with the client and how that has affected the client's behavior so far.

Observations about the client should also be included in the notes. These could be regarding the client's appearance, the way the client communicates, etc.

Mentioning any difference in the client's appearance or behavior will show whether or not the client has improved.

Finally, details about the session must be included. This could be a change in the furniture placement, a certain change of color and other objective variables that could affect a client's behavior.

Federal Laws Regarding Reporting

RBTs should be aware of federal laws surrounding reporting neglect and abuse of children. In the United States, RBTs must report to the local police and child protective services if they think a child has been neglected or abused. Further direction should be considered from a trusted supervisor.

Cases can also be reported before abuse has occurred. In these situations, the RBT can sense a possible case of abuse and report it immediately. It is necessary to report these things quickly, as such situations can become serious.

RBTs should remember in these situations that it is not their job to investigate the case. Instead, they must only report it. RBTs will not be questioned if the case is not investigated, but they can be questioned if they do not report any suspicions.

Moreover, RBTs are not in a position to ask the client if abuse or neglect has occurred. Therefore, documentation is essential and should be done professionally. This means, for example, that incident reports will need to be completed in tandem with session reports.

Handling Paperwork and Other Important Things an RBT Should Remember

Traveling with Paperwork and Storing Client Data

Paperwork that includes data collection and other essential documents must be handled according to specific laws that explain how paperwork should be stored and how an RBT should travel with paperwork.

RBTs who provide services at home need to be careful about traveling with paperwork. They must carry only necessary data. Paperwork should be stored in a briefcase and kept locked up.

RBTs are advised to speak to their supervisors about traveling with data according to the regulations provided by their workplace. All client data regarding RBT services in the United States must be stored according to Health Insurance Portability and Accountability Act (HIPAA) regulations.

According to HIPAA, client data must be stored in a secure place and should always be secured after every session. It must never be shared.

Client's Privacy

RBTs are responsible for handling the confidentiality of the client's data. Every client should be treated with respect, and one of the main ways to do this is by maintaining the confidentiality of any data collected during a session.

For any job-related communication, RBTs are required to use only relevant identifying information and not reveal information that could disclose the client's health-related data.

Even a simple conversation with another RBT about a client can violate the client's health-related data. For example, the client's name, pictures and other essential information could be used against the client by abusers. So, RBTs must remain mindful of the information they share and discuss with others.

If supervision is required for a particular case, the client and the client's family should be told about it before the client's information is shared. This should always be done for the client's best interest and the client's consent must be considered.

RBTs Supervision Documentation

RBTs are required to keep supervision documents for seven years. The BCBA can audit the supervision documentation of RBT at any time.

RBTs should have documentation ready to be presented whenever asked by the BCBA. The best way to store documentation is by scanning and saving each document electronically.

When the BCBA audits RBTs, the RBTs are given seven days to present their supervision documents. Documents held in cloud systems or online can easily be shared.

Securing Client Data

Any data relating to the client should be stored and must remain confidential. It cannot be shared with anyone, including family members. Even the most basic details must be appropriately secured. This includes session notes.

Section 6: Professional Conduct and Scope of Practice

Chapter 11: BCBA Supervision Requirements

Each RBT needs to be supervised to ensure high-quality services for future clients.

RBTs often look at supervisors as models for behavior. So, the supervisor must reflect ethical behavior. Since supervisors might be looked at as models, RBTs might adopt their habits.

A supervisor's job is to turn good RBTs into great RBTs. As supervision progresses, outcomes will be seen and improvement will be observed. Supervisors need to get a clear idea of how a certain RBT is performing, as this RBT will then be sent out in the field to work with other clients. This is why supervisors must take notes and provide timely feedback to clients for the best possible outcomes.

There are specific requirements regarding BCBA supervision. People who supervise RBTs must complete an eight-hour training based on the Supervisor Curriculum Training Outline.

The following points explain the requirements for supervision according to the Supervisor Curriculum Training Outline:

1. Stating the Purpose of Supervision

The supervisor is required to state the purpose of the supervision to the RBT. They can then supervise an RBT for several reasons, such as providing high-quality services that result in client improvement. This creates the context for clear communication and ensures the delivery's procedural fidelity.

Other reasons for supervision may include teaching the RBT conceptual skills using case examples. Supervisors also help RBTs develop decision-making skills.

2. Describing Strategies and Potential Outcomes

An RBT supervisor must be able to describe the strategies and outcomes regarding ineffective supervision, during which the supervisor will identify and discuss insufficient client progress, poor performance and unethical behavior.

Preparing Supervisory Relationship with the Trainee

The supervisor must maintain a supervisory relationship with the trainee. The Supervisor Curriculum Training Outline describes this as "determining feasible supervision capacity based on available time and resources for several activities."

These activities include maintenance of effective services, access to supervision sites in which travel time is included, preparation of content for supervision, and timely correspondence, which may consist of emails and texts.

Besides that, the supervisor must document the supervisory relationship. This documentation includes contracts and forms of supervision, work logs, background checks and documentation needed for the BCBA audit.

3. Establishing a Structured Plan

Supervisors must establish a structured plan containing supervision content and evaluation of competence for the RBT. The nature of the supervision should be reviewed.

It must include performance expectations, observation and implementation of behavioral skills training, guiding strategies, reviewed written material and an ongoing evaluation of the supervision's effects.

Structure of Supervision and Other Requirements

According to the monthly BCBA experience standards, personally developing a system for documenting supervision experience is allowed for supervisors. This makes it possible to have an individualized perspective of supervisory notes, which is acknowledged.

In addition, supervisors must complete the BCBA monthly experience and the final experience forms. No more than half of the supervision hours can be held in a group format. Supervisors must observe the RBT at least once a month with a client. The preferred way of supervision is in person; however, online observation is allowed.

As noted earlier, every RBT must obtain supervision for a minimum of 5% of the hours they spend offering services. The required amount of supervision is one hour. However, the BCBA encourages supervision of service delivery as much as possible.

How Should an RBT Be Supervised?

Supervising an RBT involves several things. Even though the supervisor needs to focus on the client's behavior toward the RBT, the focus should also be on the RBT and how he or she works with clients.

During these observations, it is essential to analyze whether or not the RBT is demonstrating appropriate behavior and communicating clearly or not. It is also crucial to determine whether the client is responding negatively or positively to the RBT.

After all of these questions are considered, the supervisor provides feedback for the RBT.

Supervision of an RBT is usually done in four steps.

- Instruction
- Demonstration
- Observation
- Feedback

The first thing a supervisor must do is instruct the RBT based on what the supervisor notices.

After the supervisor has instructed the RBT about factors that need improvement, he or she will then demonstrate how the problem can be solved.

After the demonstration is complete, the RBT will be observed while performing the particular task, keeping in mind the problems that occurred previously. The RBT will now be able to change or update the way he or she provides services according to the instruction the supervisor provided.

The supervisor will give feedback after observing the RBT for a final time. This feedback will be both verbal and in the form of notes.

Motivating Trainees

Even though giving feedback to the RBT improves his or her service-offering skills, the supervisor needs to keep track of the RBT's progress and understand that enhancing skills takes time. Therefore the RBT might not improve immediately.

The supervisor can set goals for the RBT, and feedback can be provided once the goals have been met. This will increase the chances of improvement. Supervision can sometimes be very draining for RBTs, which is why their achievements must be recognized and appreciated.

Role of RBT in Service Delivery System

An RBT must understand his or her role in the service delivery system.

The BCBA approves several credentials, such as BCBA-D, BCBA, BCaBA and RBT.

An RBT is a high school diploma-level credential.

The BCaBA is a bachelor's level credential, while the BCBA is a master's degree.

The BCBA creates a tiered service delivery model for behavior analysis services. Two organizational strategies are included in the model of service delivery. The first one includes multiple RBTs working under the direction of BCBA or BCBA-D. The other has various RBTs working under the supervision of a BCaBA and one or more BCaBAs working under the direction of a BCBA or BCBA-D.

The supervisors mentioned above are responsible for developing treatment plans, modifying treatments and providing clinical recommendations to caregivers. On the other hand, RBTs are accountable for implementing the service plans for the client and assisting some of the advisory team.

Reacting to Feedback

The reaction an RBT has toward the supervisor is critical. When the supervisor gives feedback, it becomes the RBT's responsibility to comply with it and take it seriously. If an RBT appreciates the feedback and tries to improve weak points, practical improvements would also be noticed in the client's behavior.

During the face-to-face sessions, the RBT can ask the supervisor questions related to the objective being discussed. Maintaining ethical behavior while communicating with the supervisor is essential.

RBTs should know which events require sending a self-report and which do not. The self-reporting process should be done within 30 days of an RBT becoming aware of a possibility that needs to be self-reported.

The kinds of events that require self-reporting can include legal charges against an RBT and investigations by employees, institutions and third-party payers.

Chapter 12: The Fundamentals of Professional Conduct and Scope of Practice

An RBT's behavior toward clients and clients' families should be based on kindness and respect. When conversations between an RBT and the client's family occur, the RBT must not indulge in small talk.

Small talk should also be avoided when RBTs are conversing with coworkers. This is called professional conduct, which requires RBTs to act respectfully and with consideration toward their clients.

Communication with stakeholders also has rules. RBTs are required to communicate with stakeholders only in ways they are directed. Professional boundaries and dignity must be maintained during such conversations.

Communication with Stakeholders

Stakeholders are the client's family, caregivers and other professionals. Even though RBTs do not often communicate with stakeholders, they are required to be respectful and professional when they do.

Communication between an RBT and a stakeholder can occur in several ways. Sometimes an RBT can have meetings in the form of a group with the client's family, while other times, professionals like the client's teachers and speech therapists could also be included.

An RBT needs to know the supervisor is responsible for making all clinical decisions regarding a particular case. Any questions from caregivers should pass under the purview of the supervisor.

However, the RBT should give timely input to the caregivers regarding any questions and concerns they might have. RBTs are also required to provide updates regarding the status of the ABA services.

Essential Points to Remember While Conversing with Stakeholders

Maintain Professional Conversations and Consent

RBTs must be precise and professional and avoid arguments while communicating with stakeholders. They must not discredit stakeholders' work or blame them for anything during communication.

RBTs must remember that before any conversation takes place, it is essential to have consent. Without consent, an exchange cannot be started.

Ensure Clarity and Respect

Another critical thing to ensure is that the conversation is clear and to the point. Both parties involved in the conversation must know what is being discussed. Moreover, the stakeholders must not be left out.

Some conversations might take place over the phone. In such cases, RBTs must listen to the stakeholder carefully and try not to interrupt.

Avoid Giving Unnecessary Advice

RBTs are not responsible for promising results to stakeholders. They are responsible for trying their best to help clients and provide the best services.

RBTs must not advise stakeholders regarding subjects outside their competency.

Keep Communication Logs and Providing Timely Feedback

RBTs must ensure timely feedback and maintain a communication log. When communicating with parents, RBTs must maintain reports regarding the sessions conducted with their clients and any concerns must be shared immediately.

Involving the client's family will help the client improve, and the family will also be able to analyze what can be done to help the client feel better.

Maintain Professional Boundaries

RBTs must ensure that even though they might become attached to their clients at times, they must maintain professional boundaries and act accordingly. They must never forget their role as RBTs and that they are providing professional services to a client.

RBTs must avoid any relationships with clients and stakeholders outside their professional service.

Do Not Share Your Social Media Platforms with the Client

RBTs must know that sharing the links to their social media platforms is not a healthy approach. It is also not allowed to follow a client on social media. Remember: any excessively familiar bond between the client and the RBT is prohibited.

Social media platforms reveal a person's personal life, and sharing them with a client or getting to know the client's family in this way will create a bond between the two parties that will encourage unprofessional behavior.

Do Not Accept Gifts

RBTs must not accept gifts from clients or their families. Taking gifts will get the RBT involved in a relationship outside the professional service.

Do Not Share Personal Information

While offering clients services, RBTs must ensure they do not discuss their personal issues or anything related to their personal lives with their clients or the clients' families.

Sharing such information puts the RBT in a vulnerable position and creates an emotional bond between the concerned parties. An RBT's responsibility is only to provide professional services for the client.

Sometimes the RBT might share a few personal details with clients. However, these should only be enough to maintain a friendly atmosphere and nothing more.

Avoid Exchanging Phone Numbers

Even though RBTs may sometimes provide the client's family with their phone numbers, this practice is best avoided. RBTs should be reached through their office or through email.

Exchanging phone numbers might compromise the client's and the RBT's personal information, which is a breach of law.

Personal Relationship with a Client

An RBT may only have a relationship with a former client after two years of the first service provided to the client.

Do Not Provide Services to Relatives and Family Friends

To maintain professional boundaries, RBTs must avoid working with potential clients if they know them.

Ways to Maintain Client Dignity

There are several ways to maintain a client's dignity. First, it is important to act professionally and maintain confidentiality. This is the primary way an RBT maintains the client's dignity.

However, other things must also be considered to support a client's dignity, such as:

The Client's Privacy

A client's personal information should be protected at all times. Any personal details about a client should be discussed only with the supervisor, and the information should remain within the ABA team.

Talking Down to a Client

RBTs must talk to their clients with kindness and respect. While clients must not be spoken to in an overly friendly way, they must also not be spoken to in an overly aggressive manner.

RBTs' personal beliefs must not interfere with how they treat their clients or the clients' families. For example, if an RBT dislikes smoking and notices that a client's family member smokes, the way the RBT interacts with the client must not change.

Empathy

Being empathetic toward a client is very important for RBTs. RBTs must reflect behavior that shows they care about the human in front of them, not just the money they are being paid.

Glossary

A

ABC – When a behavior occurs, RBTs must analyze the event that happened before the behavior took place using the ABC data analysis method. The behavior before the event is known as the antecedent (A). Client behavior is (B). The consequence of the behavior is (C).

Abolishing Operation – This describes antecedent events (occurring before a behavior) that momentarily decrease a consequence's reinforcing and punishing effectiveness. Due to the event, the frequency of future behavior is also altered.

Acquisition – This is the RBT's written plan, explaining behavior programming information for teaching specific skills. The plan also contains teaching strategies.

Antecedent Interventions – These are strategies designed specifically for altering the environment before a behavior occurs. This is done by modifying or removing certain elements that could be triggering a negative behavior.

Antecedent – The event before a behavior occurs is known as the antecedent.

B

Backward Chaining – This involves breaking down a task into smaller groups and working backward from the goal. The goal is the first step in this method, and backward steps reflect the factors satisfying the objective.

Behavior Intervention Plan – A BIP is a formal program that aims to stop inappropriate behavior. In this plan, the inappropriate behavior is replaced with an appropriate one. It is a therapeutic strategy used for clients.

Behavioral Skills Training – This involves instruction, modeling, rehearsal and feedback to teach a new skill. This type of training is used for instructing caregivers, parents and anyone who works with learners.

Behavior – A behavior is a range of actions and mannerisms that occur due to particular circumstances.

C

Chaining – This is a behavioral strategy used to teach students with complex behaviors. Chaining is done by breaking the behavior down into smaller, sequential steps. It is divided into forwarding and backward chaining. While forward chaining involves sequential steps toward the goal, backward chaining involves starting with the goal and moving backward.

Consequence – A consequence can be described as the result of a particular behavior. It occurs after a specific behavior has been performed. Whatever happens after a behavior can either negate or reinforce the behavior.

Continuous Measurement – This is an applied behavior analysis that measures every instance of behavior during a class, session or day.

Continuous Reinforcement – This is a form of reinforcement that involves reinforcing the client every time they perform a positive behavior.

D

Deprivation – This is the absence of the reinforcer. Deprivation in clients occurs when they have limited or no access to their reinforcer.

Differential Reinforcement – This involves reinforcing a client's positive behaviors and ignoring all others.

Discontinuous Measurement – This involves the division of observation into intervals and recording behavior that occurred during some or all of these intervals.

Discrete Trial – This is a teaching strategy that involves breaking skills down into smaller components for teaching sub-skills individually.

Discriminative Stimulus – This is a stimulus that acts as a trigger.

Dual Relationship – When RBTs are involved in multiple relationships with their clients, a dual relationship is formed. This is prohibited.

Duration – Duration involves measuring behavior and understanding how long it lasts from beginning to end.

E

Echoic – This is a form of verbal behavior that involves the speaker repeating the same sound or word said by another person.

Error Correction (ECTER) – This is a procedure in ABA that involves increasing motivation for learning situations by preventing mistakes and providing reinforcement.

Error-less Teaching – This is a form of instructional strategy that ensures clients respond correctly.

Establishing Operation – This is a motivational operation that involves the increase in the value of the reinforcer, which increases the frequency of behavior and provides access to the reinforcer.

Ethics – These are ethical codes for RBTs that describe how a client should be treated.

Expressive Language – This involves using language to communicate desires and feelings.

Extinction – This can be described as inappropriate behavior by the client, such as screaming, shouting and throwing a tantrum.

Extinction Burst – This occurs when a reinforcement that causes behavior is removed.

F

Fixed Interval – This is reinforcement done in a scheduled way. Fixed interval reinforcement occurs when a certain number of correct responses have occurred.

Forward Chaining – This is a form of reinforcement when the client is rewarded with something after completing a small task.

Frequency – Frequency is a way of measuring how many times a behavior has occurred.

Functional Behavioral Assessment – FBA is a process in which analyzed behaviors interfere with a child's learning. To avoid this, RBTs provide ways to reduce or replace those behaviors.

Functions of Behavior – In ABA, there are four functions of behavior. These include sensory stimulation, escape, access to attention and access to tangibles.

G

Generalization – This is the occurrence of a relevant behavior that happens under untrained circumstances.

H

HIPAA – This is the Health Insurance Portability and Accountability Act (HIPAA). HIPAA is a federal law that sets the national standards for protecting a person's sensitive health information.

I

Imitation – This is when someone mimics another person's behavior.

Incidental Training – In this strategy, principles of ABA are used to provide structured learning opportunities. It is done by using the client's interests and natural motivation.

Instruction Control – This involves creating a comfortable environment for clients to have them listen to the RBT.

Intermittent Reinforcement – This is a strategy in which client responses are reinforced only part of the time. In other words, reinforcement occurs in irregular intervals.

Inter-Response Time – This is the time between the end of one response and the beginning of another.

Intraverbal – This involves the speaker responding to another person's verbal behavior.

L

Latency – This records the time between the discriminative stimulus in the response.

Listener Responding – A client responding to or following directions given by others is called listener responding.

Listener Responding Feature (LRFFC) – This involves the client responding to the speaker by the feature or class of the word.

M

Magnitude – This is how the force and intensity of behavior are measured.

Maintenance – This occurs when a client's behavior continues even after teaching has ended.

Mand – This can be described as a request for something. However, the request can also be made when something is required to stop.

Measurement – This is done by measuring behavior and its intensity. In ABA, measurement can be conducted by collecting data about the client's behavior and measuring it accordingly.

Momentary Time Sample – This is a behavior assessment methodology that involves observation being divided into intervals and each interval is scored as an occurrence if the occurrence takes place at the beginning of an interval or the end.

Motivating Operation – This can be described as the motivation that encourages or discourages certain behaviors. This is done to either enhance or reduce the reinforcement value.

N

Natural Environment Teaching – This is a teaching method in which a child is taught in an environment known to him or her. The environment is something the child encounters every day.

Negative Reinforcement – This is the removal of a particular stimulus. Negative reinforcement is done as a response to a specific behavior.

O

Operational Definition – This is the process of defining behavior so it becomes measurable and observable.

P

Pairing – This is the process in which a parent is paired with the learning environment to help maintain rapport with the child.

Partial Interval Recording – This is a way of recording behavior in which the RBT marks whether a behavior occurs at any time.

Permanent Product – This is a real and concrete outcome of behavior.

Positive Reinforcement – This is reinforcement given to increase a targeted behavior.

Preference Assessment – This is an instructional tool for trainees that guides them in reinforcing a client so that the probability of the behavior can be increased.

Principles of Reinforcement (DISC) – These are the four primary personality profiles of the model of dominance, influence, steadiness and conscientiousness.

Prompt – This is assistance provided to encourage the use of a specific skill.

Prompt Hierarchy – This is the systematic structural method used to teach clients a new skill.

Prompt Fading – This is the removal of prompts paired with instruction. Prompt fading allows clients to respond correctly and independently.

Punishment – This can be described as the decrease in the occurrence of specific behavior resulting from an event that followed the behavior.

R

Rate – This is the measurement of behavior, calculating the number of times a behavior occurs during an interval.

Reactive Strategies – This is a strategic method that involves establishing control over a situation to minimize the risk associated with behavior. This is done by bringing out immediate behavioral change in a client.

Receptive Language – This is the understanding of provided information in different ways, including words, sounds and gestures.

Reinforcement – This is a reward given to a client after a specific behavior.

Replacement Behavior – This involves replacing behaviors that limit a client's learning process with behaviors that encourage learning.

Response Prompt – This is assistance for evoking a correct response in an individual through verbal, modeling and physical guidance.

Role of RBT – The role of the RBT is the different ways he or she can work and perform.

S

Satiation – This is an ABA principle that says that too much of any good thing will result in that thing not being preferred anymore.

Secondary Reinforcers – These reinforcers need to be learned through pairings with unconditioned reinforcers. Money is an example.

Setting Events – These are the events concurring before a behavior.

Shaping – This is the reinforcement of successive approximations of the desired behavior.

Skill Acquisition – This is a plan that includes teaching strategies and a description of the skill being taught to the client.

Spontaneous Recovery – This is the fading away of a particular behavior even after reinforcement. This is the reappearance of the conditioned recovery response after a period of rest.

Stimulus – This is a change in energy that affects an organism through the receptor cells. A stimulus often results in behavior.

Stimulus Control – This involves controlling specific triggers that result in particular behaviors.

Stimulus Control Transfer – This is a technique that involves the discontinuation of prompts once the target behavior is achieved.

Stimulus Prompt – This makes the discriminative stimulus target behavior prominent.

T

Tact – This is a form of verbal behavior that occurs when the speaker comments about something they see, hear or smell.

Task Analysis – This breaks down complex tasks into more minor sequences or actions.

Token Economy – These are economies based on the principles of ABA that emphasize using positive reinforcement for behavioral change.

Topography – This is the descriptive way in which a behavior is analyzed. Topography describes the way a behavior looks.

V

Variable Interval – This is a schedule of reinforcement that records the first correct response following an average amount of predetermined time.

Variable Ratio – This is a schedule reinforcement that involves delivering a reinforcer after an average number of responses have occurred.

W

Whole Interval Recording – This is the recording of behavior that occurs during the entire interval.

Test 1

Section 1: Measurement

(1) The horizontal line at the bottom of the graph, known as the _________, signifies the passage of time. The vertical line on the graph's left is called the ______________.

(A) y-axis; x-axis.

(B) x-axis; condition.

(C) x-axis; condition.

(D) x-axis; y-axis.

(2) During snack break, Joshua chewed his food for two minutes, sang for five minutes and looked out the window for two minutes.

What can an RBT measure in this scenario?

(A) Latency.

(B) Rate.

(C) Inter-response time.

(D) Duration.

(3) Observing a behavior for a fixed amount of time, such as five minutes, and then reporting if the target behavior occurred at any point during your observation is required for a discontinuous data collection technique known as __________.

(A) Partial interval recording.

(B) Whole interval recording.

(C) Latency data recording.

(D) Momentary time sampling.

(4) ________ is a type of data collection that records things such as clean dishes on a drying rack, an empty trash can in the house and a beautifully made bed.

(A) Continuous measurement.

(B) Permanent product recording.

(C) Frequency.

(D) Mastered target.

(5) Mike is a client you work with as an RBT. Your BCBA directs you to collect data on Mike staying with his mom during grocery shopping without straying away. You are told to use the whole interval recording approach with two-minute intervals.

How would you capture the information?

(A) Record the behavior using a + if Mike stayed with his mom at any point during the two-minute interval.

(B) Record the behavior using a - if Mike was with his mom at the end of the two-minute interval.

(C) Record the number of times (frequency) Mike left his mom during the two-minute interval.

(D) Record the behavior using + if Mike stayed with his mom for the entire two-minute interval.

(6) Which of the following behaviors is the most measurable and observable by definition?

(A) Peter frequently acts out of control.

(B) Peter responds to perceived taunts from others because he thinks they are trying to harm him.

(C) Peter irritates people by poking them with his finger.

(D) Peter suffers from an intermittent explosive disorder contributing to his aggressive outbursts.

(7) Jennifer, an RBT, will gather information about Lily, a preschooler, and her tendency to bite nails. She chooses to record events at four-minute intervals. Jennifer defines nail biting as when Lily puts her fingers in her mouth to bite her nails. She records the behavior on the datasheet for a one-minute interval if Lily exhibits nail biting at any point.

Jenny is employing _________.

(A) Momentary time sampling.

(B) Partial time sampling.

(C) Permanent product recording.

(D) Whole interval recording.

(8) For which of the following will permanent-product procedures be most suitable?

(A) Measuring how frequently students behave aggressively toward others.

(B) Determining whether Michael purchases all the food items on his shopping list.

(C) Calculating how long it takes a toddler to put on his shoes after the initial instruction.

(D) Identifying self-destructive behavior.

(9) Which discontinuous measurement is the most direct and conservative way to monitor a student's participation in a lesson?

(A) Interviewing the teacher.

(B) Partial interval recording.

(C) Momentary time sampling.

(D) Whole interval recording.

(10) Preparation to gather data entails several steps. Which of the following would the RBT perform first?

(A) Verifying data.

(B) Choosing the right measuring strategy.

(C) Gathering baseline data.

(D) Defining the target behavior.

(11) What type of graph is mostly used to visually analyze the recordings of permanent- product procedures?

(A) Line graph.

(B) Parabola.

(C) Bar graph.

(D) Pie chart.

(12) Good (credible) data collection is integral to ABA. Which of the following are signs of good data?

(A) Reliable, accurate and valid data.

(B) Verified data.

(C) Scientifically proven data.

(D) Hypsographical accurate data.

Section 2: Assessment

(13) Identifying activities or events that come before a behavior, describing the actions that are observed and denoting the actions that immediately follow a response is a type of data collection method known as __________.

(A) Partial interval recording.

(B) Antecedent intervention.

(C) Latency recording.

(D) ABC data collection.

(14) What is the aim and purpose of stimulus preferences?

(A) They act as test motivators (reinforcers) for the client.

(B) They help the RBT decide what actions or things will constitute negative reinforcement for a client.

(C) They recognize potential stimulating items, places or activities.

(D) They help clients select the intervention they prefer.

(15) You can be asked to help with functional assessments as an RBT. Your participation will most likely be through indirect measures.

What will these measures include?

(A) Functional manipulation in viva.

(B) Functional manipulation in analog settings.

(C) Observation and preference data collection on a topic.

(D) Performing interviews, surveys and creating rating scales.

(16) Rosa performed a preference assessment for Daisy, a six-year-old autistic girl. Before the assessment, Rosa allowed her to play with the eight stimuli set out on a table. Rosa then began her assessment. She set aside the first item when Daisy picked it. Then she noticed which item Daisy selected next. After that, Rosa set aside the next object when Daisy selected it.

What classification of preference assessment did Rosa conduct?

(A) Single-stimulus preference assessment.

(B) Paired-stimulus preference assessment.

(C) Multiple-stimulus preference assessment with replacement.

(D) Multiple-stimulus preference assessment without replacement.

(17) A method for determining possible stimuli preferences includes:

(A) Determining what the client enjoys.

(B) Finding out from others what the client likes.

(C) Understanding subjects' preferences by seeing them in their natural environment.

(D) Using a published list of things or activities that children enjoy.

(18) You are working with Gina, a 16-year-old girl. You think that Gina might find reinforcement in food. She does not have any dietary or health constraints. You decide to test her preference for potato chips versus nuts and fruits.

You simultaneously provide Gina with a choice between a jar of nuts and a bag of potato chips. Gina decides to go with the nut jar. Then you give her the option of a jar of nuts and a bowl of mixed fruit together. She chooses the nut jar once again.

What kind of assessment did you carry out?

(A) Free-operant observation preference assessment.

(B) Single-stimulus preference assessment.

(C) Forced-choice preference assessment.

(D) Multiple-stimulus preference assessment without replacement.

Section 3: Skill Acquisition

(19) A behavior analyst develops a written plan that includes details of behavior programming to teach skills.

What is this method called?

(A) Master plan.

(B) Skill acquisition plan.

(C) General plan.

(D) Maintenance plan.

(20) Which of the following best describes the importance of data for behavior analysts?

(A) It helps them evaluate the learner's development.

(B) It helps them understand response patterns.

(C) It helps them determine how to change strategies.

(D) It helps them promote student independence.

(21) Collected data can be used to identify response patterns. What is an example of a response pattern?

(A) An increase or decrease in target behaviors.

(B) The effectiveness of instructional methods.

(C) Student independence.

(D) Teaching new skills.

(22) John is a behavior analyst who collects human behavior data that contains information on preferences, beliefs and attitudes.

Which of the following best describes how John collects data?

(A) Surveys.

(B) Interviews.

(C) Observational data.

(D) Demographic data.

(23) ______ can be used to acquire information about age, gender, ethnicity and socioeconomic status.

(A) Demographic data.

(B) Observational data.

(C) Discrete data.

(D) Astrographic data.

(24) Which of the following best describes comprehending consumer behavior and targeting products and services to specific audiences?

(A) Government policies.

(B) Public policy.

(C) Interviews.

(D) Market research.

(25) Which list below contains essential elements found in RBTs' work?

(A) Frequency data, duration data, partial interval, whole interval and permanent products.

(B) Frequency data, duration data, public policy, whole interval and mental health.

(C) Frequency data, government policymaking, public policy, whole interval and permanent products.

(D) Observational data, government policymaking, public policy, whole interval and permanent products.

(26) ________ describes how often a behavior occurs within a given time frame.

(A) Duration data.

(B) Partial interval.

(C) Frequency data.

(D) Whole interval.

(27) Which of the following best describes the length of time a behavior occurs?

(A) Duration data.

(B) Partial interval.

(C) Frequency data.

(D) Whole interval.

(28) Which data component can be used to acquire information about tangible outcomes of particular behaviors?

(A) Duration data.

(B) Partial interval.

(C) Frequency data.

(D) Permanent products.

(29) Which of the following best describes what a scatterplot shows?

(A) Recording the occurrence of a particular behavior over an extended period.

(B) A target behavior that occurs for the complete duration of a specific period.

(C) The length of time of behavior occurs.

(D) How often a behavior occurs within a given time frame.

(30) Which list below contains a procedure that needs to be followed for achieving skill objectives described by ABA using a common perspective language?

(A) Presentation, description, error correction, reinforcement and plan for reinforcement.

(B) Presentation, description, public policy, reinforcement and plan for reinforcement.

(C) Presentation, instructions, SR +/- and error correction.

(D) Presentation, description, error correction, reinforcement and plan for reinforcement.

(31) Which of the following best describes target behavior?

(A) A reaction that resembles a model of the trainer and occurs within three seconds.

(B) When clients complete their skill goals.

(C) An objective that reflects the development of a skill.

(D) A skill that needs to be learned.

(32) Which list below contains essential components of the behavior goal?

(A) A description of desired behavior, techniques for gathering data, skill acquisition.

(B) A description of circumstance under which conduct takes place, description of desired behavior, description of requirements for success.

(C) A description of desired behavior, reactionary techniques, presentation.

(D) A description of desired behavior, techniques for gathering data, permanent products.

(33) How can the term *learning strategy* be best defined?

(A) Teaching a child with ASD categories.

(B) Materials consistent with teaching materials.

(C) Activities that assist students in achieving their learning objectives.

(D) Managing a treatment program that leads to positive reinforcement.

(34) What are some phrases that can be used to define *action* in learning techniques?

(A) Review, describe and fact.

(B) Discover, learn and experiential.

(C) Teach, learn and review.

(D) Construct, reflexivity and learn.

(35) ________ describes a structured sequence of activities to support a learner's development from fundamental to advanced skill acquisition.

(A) Naturalistic teaching.

(B) Plan strategy.

(C) Skill acquisition.

(D) Task analysis.

(36) Derek uses a technique that allows him to reinforce a specific healthy behavior while avoiding undesirable behaviors.

What is this technique called?

(A) Behavioral analysis.

(B) Contingent reinforcement.

(C) Naturalistic teaching.

(D) Fixation.

(37) How can response cues be administered?

(A) Orally, through modeling or physically.

(B) Orally, through modeling or naturally.

(C) Orally, through modeling or artificially.

(D) Regularly, through modeling or artificially.

(38) Normal reinforcement is improved by using another reinforcer, such as tokens, praises, grades, etc.

What is this type of reinforcement called?

(A) Unconditioned reinforcement.

(B) Conditioned reinforcement.

(C) Intermittent reinforcement.

(D) Regular reinforcement.

(39) A child is given a favorite toy after completing a task. This is an example of _________.

(A) Positive reinforcement.

(B) Negative reinforcement.

(C) Neither positive nor negative reinforcement.

(D) All of the above.

(40) A mother removes the punishment of doing additional homework because her child obtained good grades at school. This is an example of _______.

(A) Negative enforcement.

(B) Positive Enforcement.

(C) Maintaining neutrality.

(D) None of the above.

(41) Which of the following lists contains different types of schedules of reinforcement?

(A) Fixed ratio, regular interval, variable ratio, variable interval.

(B) Fixed ratio, fixed interval, variable ratio, variable interval.

(C) Fixed ratio, regular interval, variable ratio, fixed interval.

(D) Fixed ratio, fixed interval, physical ratio, variable interval.

(42) On average, every five bites of cauliflower results in a bite of burger for a child working with an RBT. Which reinforcement is used in the example?

(A) Fixed ratio.

(B) Variable interval.

(C) Variable ratio.

(D) Fixed interval.

Section 4: Behavior Reduction

(43) What are the four functions of behavior?

(A) Toys, edibles, praise and aversion.

(B) Escape, sensory, tangibles and attention.

(C) Sensory overload, noncompliance, aggression and compliance.

(D) Automatic sensory, automatic positive, neutral negative and social negative.

(44) Amber stays in her room for several hours to avoid interacting with anyone. This could be an example of __________.

(A) Sensory stimulation.

(B) Anger management.

(C) Escapist behavior.

(D) Access to attention.

(45) Which of the following is used to measure behavior?

(A) Reaction analysis.

(B) RBT notes.

(C) Real-time observation.

(D) Both (A) and (C).

(46) What impact does reinforcement have on behavior?

(A) It has a negative effect.

(B) It plays no role.

(C) It positively increases the future behavioral outlook.

(D) None of the above.

(47) What is the function of visual timers?

(A) They aid RBTs in timing when to transition.

(B) They show photos of transitioning.

(C) They help with communication.

(D) Both (A) and (C).

(48) Which of the following best describes replacement behavior?

(A) Following the same behavior.

(B) An easier and temporary replacement behavior.

(C) A long-term behavior for a permanent solution.

(D) An unhealthy and complex alternative.

(49) What is differential reinforcement?

(A) Encouragement of positive behavior.

(B) Highlighting negative aspects.

(C) Ignoring all behavior.

(D) Punishment.

(50) Neutral redirection can put a stop to all problematic behavioral issues. Is this true?

(A) Yes. It can remove issues immediately by providing extra attention.

(B) No. It can stop aggressive behaviors only by shifting to others.

(C) No. It cannot control any behavior.

(D) Yes. It can get rid of specific issues but in a reckless manner.

(51) How do experts identify why a behavior occurs?

(A) By analyzing essential behavioral functions.

(B) By looking at sensory stimulation.

(C) By the client's actions.

(D) None of the above.

(52) __________ is an example of sensory stimulation.

(A) Running away.

(B) Scratching skin.

(C) Screaming aggressively.

(D) Ignoring everyone.

(53) How many functions of behavior are present in ABA therapy?

(A) Four.

(B) Three.

(C) Two.

(D) One.

(54) Jared is struggling with his mental health. He constantly throws tantrums and displays aggressive behavior.

What are the necessary steps an RBT must follow when interacting with Jared?

(A) Offer Jared positive reinforcement.

(B) Wear normal clothes.

(C) Wear extra protective equipment and proceed with care.

(D) Entertain Jared with personal anecdotes.

Section 5: Documentation and Reporting

(55) If an RBT is asked to do something she has no knowledge about, what should she do?

(A) Try it out, then ask the supervisor.

(B) Immediately ask the supervisor for assistance and guidance.

(C) Read the guidebook and see if she can manage.

(D) Document the request without interrupting the session and talk to the supervisor later.

(56) Helga completed her session under the BCBA's supervision. She kept track of the session's data on a paper data collection sheet. However, she accidentally ruined her data sheet by spilling a cup of coffee all over it, rendering it unreadable.

How should Helga proceed? Her organization has tough standards when it comes to employees who do not correctly submit data at the end of a shift.

(A) Helga should not tell anybody what happened and hope that nobody notices the missing session notes.

(B) Helga should estimate the client's proficiency with each skill target. Since it was not all that long ago, she probably remembers everything without any problems.

(C) Helga should report the incident to her supervisor and work to avoid a similar mishap in the future, perhaps by implementing mechanical or digital data collection systems.

(D) During the subsequent supervision meeting, Helga should give her supervisor the coffee-stained paper data sheet and resign.

(57) A client who is typically enthusiastic and willing to work is being assisted by an RBT. However, the client is currently acting unwell and would rather lie on the floor than sit on a chair.

What should the RBT do?

(A) Ask the client what is wrong and offer help.

(B) Conduct the session while sitting on the floor.

(C) Tell the supervisor or family right away about the client's behavior and condition.

(D) Postpone the session until the client feels better.

(58) Which of the following terms is used for avoiding dual relationships, conflicts of interest and social media contacts with clients?

(A) Maintaining professional boundaries.

(B) Working through the ADA method.

(C) Maintaining competency.

(D) Ensuring the ADRCC.

(59) Which of the following phrases would be best for a session note with an objective?

(A) "Today, during mand training and visual discrimination, Katia did well."

(B) "Sienna underperformed during training."

(C) "Hawke completed the handwashing procedure step by step on his own."

(D) "Zoe needed a lot of encouragement today to finish the majority of her assignments."

(60) What does it mean when RBTs are asked to use feedback and reflection?

(A) They are asked to respond appropriately to feedback and maintain or improve their performance.

(B) They are asked to take feedback and work as reflective practitioners.

(C) They are asked to behave professionally.

(D) All of the above.

(61) Which of the following approaches is ideal for maintaining the confidentiality of session records in writing?

(A) Not making any notes.

(B) Storing the scanned copy of the document in an encrypted file and scrapping the written documents.

(C) Putting the notes in a file folder and locking them in a filing cabinet.

(D) Recording sessions in RBT code words and acronyms.

(62) In the service delivery system, the role of the RBT involves ________.

(A) Maintaining a professional demeanor when practicing in the designated area under direct observation.

(B) Implementing measurement, evaluation, skill development and behavior reduction.

(C) Data collection, reporting and documentation.

(D) All of the above.

(63) Records and information gathered by BCBAs and RBTs must be kept for at least _____ years, in addition to any other time periods specified by law.

(A) Seven.

(B) Six.

(C) Five.

(D) Four.

(64) An RBT should document _______.

(A) Real-time observations.

(B) Interpretations of what was observed.

(C) Variables that might affect the client.

(D) Both (A) and (C).

Section 6: Professional Conduct and Scope of Practice

(65) Which of the following processes ensures optimum quality of services for an RBT's future clients?

(A) Supervision.

(B) Training.

(C) Services.

(D) Supportive environment.

(66) Regarding professional conduct, RBTs should avoid ______ when conversing with clients, clients' families and coworkers.

(A) Kindness.

(B) Communication.

(C) Respect.

(D) Small talk.

(67) "Determining feasible supervision capacity based on available time and resources for several activities."

This defines a _________.

(A) Supervisory relationship.

(B) Structured relationship.

(C) Trainee relationship.

(D) General relationship.

(68) Why must RBTs not accept gifts from clients or clients' families?

(A) It is a sign of disrespect.

(B) It will lead to RBTs engaging in a relationship outside their professional area.

(C) It can have legal consequences.

(D) It is not allowed.

(69) How many maximum supervision hours can be held in a session format?

(A) 1/2 of the supervision hours.

(B) 1/4 of supervision hours.

(C) 1/3 of supervision hours.

(D) 1/5 of supervision hours.

(70) Which of the following lists contains the requirements for supervision according to the Supervisor Curriculum Training Outline?

(A) Initiating the purpose of supervision, describing strategies and outcomes, enlisting in behavioral training and making a structured plan.

(B) Initiating the purpose of supervision, describing strategies and outcomes, entering a supervisory relationship with the teacher and making a structured plan.

(C) Initiating the purpose of behavioral training, describing strategies and outcomes, entering a supervisory relationship with the trainee and making a structured plan.

(D) Initiating the purpose of supervision, describing strategies and outcomes, entering a supervisory relationship with the trainee and making a structured plan.

(71) An RBT intends to provide the client's family with their phone number. Why should the client's family not accept the RBT's phone number?

(A) It can compromise the RBT's and client's personal information.

(B) It is illegal.

(C) It will affect the supervision plan.

(D) It increases the time for supervision.

(72) What are the four steps for the supervision of an RBT?

(A) Instruction, demonstration, observation and feedback.

(B) Instruction, behavioral training, observation and feedback.

(C) Instruction, behavioral training, client training and feedback.

(D) General training, behavioral training, observation and feedback.

(73) When is it permissible for an RBT to maintain a relationship with a former client?

(A) This is allowed two years after the first service is provided to a client.

(B) It is permissible at any time.

(C) It is not permissible.

(D) None of the above.

(74) Why should RBTs avoid working with their relatives or family friends?

(A) Because RBTs may form an emotional bond with their clients, which can impact their workflow.

(B) Because it would be a conflict of interest.

(C) Because RBTs are not encouraged to work with their relatives or family friends.

(D) Because it is against the law.

(75) Why must supervisors encourage and appreciate the achievements of RBTs?

(A) Supervision can be exhausting for RBTs, so their achievements need to be appreciated.

(B) Supervisors are discouraged from appreciating the achievements of RBTs.

(C) Supervisors are legally not allowed to appreciate RBTs' achievements.

(D) It is required by the law.

(76) An RBT observes a client's vocal stimming behaviors during a session. The RBT decides to record the frequency of this behavior. Which method of data collection is most appropriate during the session?

(A) Duration recording.

(B) Frequency recording.

(C) Partial interval recording.

(D) Momentary time sampling.

(77) An RBT needs to measure how long it takes a client to respond to a given instruction. Which data collection method should they use?

(A) Latency recording.

(B) Interval recording.

(C) Frequency recording.

(D) Permanent product recording.

(78) In a classroom, an RBT observes a client's behavior when they raise a hand to answer questions. The behavior and its occurrences are to be measured over one hour. Which data collection method would be best?

(A) Whole interval recording.

(B) Partial interval recording.

(C) Momentary time sampling.

(D) Frequency recording.

(79) An RBT evaluates a client's progress in independently completing assigned tasks. The outcome is tangible and can be observed after the session. Which method of data collection should be used?

(A) Duration recording.

(B) Frequency recording.

(C) Permanent product recording.

(D) Latency recording.

(80) To assess the effectiveness of a new intervention strategy, an RBT decides to track a specific behavior's occurrence over several weeks. The goal is to identify trends and changes in the behavior's frequency over time. Which graphical representation would best illustrate these changes?

(A) Pie chart.

(B) Bar graph.

(C) Line graph.

(D) Scatter plot.

(81) An RBT works with a twelve-year-old girl who is selectively mute in social settings and shows interest in drawing and music. The goal is to increase her verbal communication. Which preference assessment method would best identify activities that could encourage verbal responses?

(A) Free-operant observations.

(B) Single stimulus.

(C) Paired stimulus.

(D) Multiple stimulus without replacement.

(82) A fifteen-year-old boy with autism spectrum disorder is observed to have several preferences that change frequently. To maintain his interest in skill acquisition programs, how should the RBT proceed with preference assessments?

(A) Conduct a single stimulus preference assessment weekly.

(B) Use a multiple stimulus with replacement assessment daily.

(C) Perform a paired stimulus preference assessment monthly.

(D) Implement free-operant observations throughout the day.

(83) An eight-year-old child shows aggressive behavior when asked to transition between activities. An RBT plans to use preference assessments to identify reinforcers that could facilitate smoother transitions. What type of preference assessment might pose the least risk of aggressive behavior?

(A) Multiple stimulus without replacement.

(B) Paired stimulus.

(C) Single stimulus.

(D) Free-operant observations.

(84) In a case where a client demonstrates difficulty when they make choices between more than two options, which preference assessment method is most appropriate to identify potential reinforcers?

(A) Paired stimulus.

(B) Multiple stimulus with replacement.

(C) Single stimulus.

(D) Multiple stimulus without replacement.

(85) A client has shown a significant improvement in appropriate behaviors when highly preferred items are presented as rewards. However, the RBT noticed a plateau in their progress. To enhance the client's motivation and skill acquisition, what strategy should they consider in the context of preference assessments?

(A) Rotate between different types of preference assessments weekly.

(B) Introduce novel stimuli in a free-operant observation setting.

(C) Increase the frequency of multiple stimulus without replacement assessments.

(D) Conduct an indirect functional assessment to explore new interests.

Test 1: Answers and Explanations

Section 1: Measurement

(1) (D) x-axis; y-axis.

The horizontal axis is called the x-axis, and the y-axis is the vertical axis. The x-axis measures the independent variable, and the y-axis measures the dependent variable. Usually the dependent variable shows the data of the behavior being measured.

(2) (D) Duration.

Duration recording measures the length of time a pupil exhibits a particular behavior. In this case, the durations of each activity, such as chewing, singing and looking out of the window, are two, five and two minutes respectively.

The length of time between an antecedent (such as a teacher's instruction) and the moment the student starts to carry out a certain behavior is measured by latency recording.

Inter-response time is the period between two instances of an activity that occur back to back. The frequency of the behavior in an amount of time is referred to as its rate.

(3) (A) Partial interval recording.

When documenting partial intervals, the observer notes if a behavior occurred at any point in the interval. A sample of the prescribed behavior at the precise moment that data is being collected is known as momentary time sampling.

When the observer is interested in behavior that takes place during the full interval, it is called whole interval recording. Latency recording is a type of continuous measurement that measures the time between an antecedent (such as a teacher's instruction) and the moment the student starts to carry out a certain behavior.

(4) (B) Permanent-product recording.

Permanent-product recording is a type of measurement in which a product or outcome that signifies the existence of the target or replacement behavior is chosen. The response is recorded depending on whether the product is generated or not.

RBTs should not use this technique as their main method of gathering data.

(5) (D) Record the behavior using + if Mike stayed with his mom for the entire two-minute interval.

You can use whole interval recording to check if the client's behavior continues without interruption during the given interval. You may count the number of intervals in which the behavior occurred throughout the entire interval.

In this case, you record if Mike stayed with his mom throughout the two-minute intervals. Later, you may count the two-minute intervals in which Mike stayed with his mom throughout.

(6) (C) Peter irritates people by poking them with his finger.

Poking somebody in the arm with a finger is an observable and quantifiable quantity.

Behavior that is out of control or expressed in other verbal ways cannot be observed or measured. In Option A, the number of suspensions is quantifiable (they may be regarded as permanent products), but the conduct is not. Instead, the RBT gauges how people react to the conduct(s).

Option B does not define the behavior but rather provides a potential antecedent or trigger for it. It uses a diagnostic label to describe behavior, which is a supposition and frequently more detrimental than beneficial. If described in more detail, aggressive outbursts may be observable and measurable.

(7) (B) Partial time sampling.

In partial time sampling, a behavior is displayed at least once throughout the defined interval to be considered to have happened. In contrast, the behavior is recorded as a whole interval if it occurred throughout the interval without any break.

(8) (B) Determining whether Michael purchases all the food items on his shopping list.

Permanent-product procedures track the material outcomes of behavior; these also include the effect caused on the environment. So, the RBT must concentrate on assessing the end product of an observation rather than the process of creating permanent product recording techniques.

The quantity of words a student records in a two-minute session may become a final product. The product could be checked after the activity has taken place by recording if all of the groceries on Michael's list were bought. Other examples of a permanent product include completed worksheets, solved puzzles or properly made beds.

(9) (D) Whole interval recording.

A direct measurement involves actual observation. In contrast, indirect measurements include observations of others, like a checklist, interview or rating scale. The most suitable discontinuous measurement would be whole interval recording. Because it is applied to activities that endure longer, it would provide the most reliable information.

When recording whole intervals, the behavior must take place for the entire interval to be recorded as an occurrence. For example, in whole interval recording, the RBT would record if the student paid attention in class for the entire predefined interval.

(10) (D) Defining the target behavior.

The first step of measuring data is to define the data being measured/the target behavior. Data collection and analysis are essential to ABA. To understand how behaviors function, clinicians and practitioners require data. It allows them to formulate hypotheses and design intervention tactics.

(11) (C) Bar graphs.

A bar graph might be the most appropriate option when comparing final products in permanent-product procedures. This is because end products are tangible and measured as whole numbers.

A bar chart is one of the best options for comparing multiple values within the same subject. Using a bar chart, the RBT can show how a client's behavior has improved and determine whether any significant changes need to be looked at to ensure the client receives the best possible care.

On the other hand, a pie chart is perfect for classifying data because each slice or segment on the graph corresponds to a certain category. It might also be appropriate for describing and contrasting various target behaviors.

(12) (A) Reliable, accurate and valid data.

In applied behavior analysis, we aim to gather believable data which is extremely accurate, reliable and valid data. The validity and accuracy of data can be confirmed through frequent collections and constant verification.

Verification is done after collecting data to ensure we are measuring what we should be measuring.

Section 2: Assessment

(13) (D) ABC data collection.

Antecedent, behavior and consequence (ABC) recording is a method of gathering data to assist in identifying the purpose of a client's behavior.

It accomplishes this goal by dividing observations into three categories: antecedents (A) or the events that occurred immediately before the behavior, the particular action(s) or behavior of interest (B) and the consequence (C) or action that happened after the behavior (B).

The antecedent recording is a part of ABC recording. Latency recording is a type of continuous measurement that refers to the time between instruction and response.

Partial interval recording is a type of discontinuous data collection in which you check if a behavior occurred in a specific interval.

(14) (C) They recognize potential stimulating items, places or activities.

When and where a person favors a particular stimulus is revealed through stimulus preference assessments, along with the stimuli preferred and the relative value of each stimulus.

(15) (D) Performing interviews, surveys and creating rating scales.

As an RBT, you observe behavior through direct and indirect assessment. In an indirect assessment method, you do not directly observe the client's behavior; instead, you use various types of indirect assessment to assemble background data.

These methods may include interviewing caretakers and guardians, creating systematic rating systems and creating questionnaires.

(16) (D) Multiple-stimulus preference assessment without replacement.

A collection of items known as the array is the basis of the multiple-stimulus preference assessment without replacement. The items that need to be put in an array must first be identified by the RBT. Although there is no predetermined number, a reasonable array contains roughly six to eight items.

While working with clients, an RBT presents them with an array of items (often toys or sweets) and asks them to choose one. The RBT takes the item out of the collection after the client uses or consumes it. After that, the RBT notes items in the array and the client's choice of each item.

(17) (D) Using a published list of things or activities that children enjoy.

A stimulus preference assessment does not determine reinforcers; instead, it identifies the things, people or activities that could reinforce a behavior. It does this by querying others, free-operant observation and trial-based evaluations such as forced choice.

Other methods to determine probable favorite stimuli may include presenting a person with various options to choose from or ranking certain items to measure preference relatively. The information acquired from these assessments could subsequently be used in situations to verify that certain stimuli are, in fact, reinforcements. The same procedure can also be used to find potential punishers.

(18) (C) Forced-choice preference assessment.

Forced-choice preference assessment means providing a choice between two options. In this case, you have found that the jar of nuts actually has the greatest potential as a reinforcer by conducting a forced-choice preference assessment.

Sometimes only a few things are used in stimulus preference tests, while other times, a client is offered a selection of, say, eight items and asked to choose one. This is how a preference analysis is carried out.

The terms *with replacement* and *without replacement* refer to whether you add the client-selected item back to the array or move forward without it (the client picking from seven toys in the example).

Section 3: Skill Acquisition

(19) (B) Skill acquisition plan.

A skill acquisition plan is a plan written by a behavior analyst. It contains information relevant to behavior programming.

Skill acquisition plans include a description of skills being taught and appropriate teaching materials. These plans consist of mastery criteria, reinforcement techniques and a generalization and maintenance plan.

(20) (A) It helps them evaluate the learner's development.

RBTs are responsible for continuously assessing learners' development. They record extensive information about learners' behavior and determine if they are remaining stagnant, becoming worse or growing better by receiving accurate feedback on their performance.

(21) (A) An increase or decrease in target behaviors.

RBTs can analyze data collected to identify relevant response patterns. An example of a response pattern is an increase or decrease in target behaviors.

(22) (A) Surveys.

Behavior analysts use different types of data to comprehend human behavior. Surveys, interviews, observational data and demographics are standard data collection methods. Survey data contains information on beliefs, preferences and attitudes.

Observation data includes information about body language, facial expressions and how humans interact with each other. In contrast, demographic data can be about age, ethnicity, gender and socioeconomic status.

(23) (A) Demographic data.

Behavior analysts use demographic data to understand human behavior through gender, ethnicity, age and socioeconomic status. Demographic data represents the socioeconomic information displayed statistically, including education, employment, marriage rates, mortality rate, etc.

Businesses often use demographic data as a marketing tool to determine the optimum method to reach customers and evaluate their behavior.

(24) (D) Market research.

Market research refers to businesses comprehending consumer behavior and better targeting their products and services to their audiences. It is the process whereby businesses determine the viability of a new product or service through research conducted directly with the consumers.

(25) (A) Frequency data, duration data, partial interval, whole interval and permanent products.

Data components used by RBTs include frequency data, duration data, partial data, whole interval and permanent products. This information is essential to show the participant's behavior has changed.

Frequency data refers to how often the behavior occurs within a time frame. It must have a clear start and stop. In contrast, duration data refers to the length of time for a behavior to occur while the time measurement is specified.

When target behavior occurs for a part of a specified period, it is known as a partial interval. The whole interval refers to when the target behavior occurs for the complete duration of a specified period.

(26) (C) Frequency data.

Frequency data involves recording the number of times a behavior happens in a given time frame. The behavior needs to have a clear start and stop. An example could be the number of times a child bangs a fist against the desk or how many students write on desks.

This type of data can help behavior analysts evaluate how problematic an issue is and determine the best action needed for solving a specific behavioral problem. Frequency data is helpful only when the behavioral event has a clear beginning and end.

Behavior analysts can use frequency data with behaviors that cannot be measured precisely. For instance, if a child gets aggressive for only half an hour, you cannot count how many times the child gets aggressive in a three-hour time frame.

So, to measure frequency data, you can set up a time frame where you will measure the behavior. When the first behavior happens, you can note the time and tally each behavioral fluctuation according to the time frame.

(27) (A) Duration data.

Duration data is the length of time a behavior occurs and provides the time measurement. Behavioral analysts use it to document the amount of time a student spends engaging in a behavior.

Using duration data, analysts can observe the behavior with a clear start and end. Instances of behavior could be reading a book, crying, writing in class, etc. Wall clocks, wristwatches and stopwatches are some instruments analysts use to record the duration of a behavior.

(28) (D) Permanent products.

Permanent products are real or tangible outcomes that result from a behavior. They look at behavior that results in lasting outcomes.

For example, a teacher may be interested in how well a student cleans up after an art activity. The identified behavior is removing pieces of paper and debris from the desk. A permanent product outcome could be counting paper pieces that remain on the desk after the student has finished cleaning up.

(29) (A) Recording the occurrence of a particular behavior over an extended period.

A scatterplot refers to recording the occurrence of behavior over an extended time frame. It reflects a pattern that may be concerned with any event related to a specific time.

Usually, a scatterplot visually represents a problem behavior by the time of day at which it occurs. It can help the behavioral analyst identify times of a day that may be concerned with high or low rates of problem behavior.

A scatterplot is a grid with time plotted on the vertical line divided into different time frames. The time listed on the grid might be divided into 20-minute periods. The first time on the grid could be 10:00 to 10:20 and the next could be 10:20 to 10:40.

In some situations, it may be helpful to use a 30-minute or one-hour time frame, depending on the type of behavior and length of time you are observing. Different time frames allow behavioral analysts to identify when problem behaviors may occur.

The advantage of a scatterplot includes that several strategies can be used, including duration, latency and frequency data. Moreover, the exact number of behaviors can be written into cells to provide more extensive information.

(30) (C) Presentation, instructions, SR +/- and error correction.

A skill acquisition plan must be well written and include a detailed description of the steps. The procedure that the analysts implement to achieve skill objectives is identified by ABA using a common perspective language.

The measures include presentation, instructions, reinforcement, plan for reinforcement and error correction. Presentation is a way of teaching and instructions refer to the intended response. SR +/- is reinforcement and strategy for support, while error correction refers to correcting errors.

(31) (A) A reaction that resembles a model of the trainer and occurs within three seconds.

The target behavior is a reaction that resembles the trainer's model and occurs within three seconds. The behavior includes all observable actions taken by a living organism. It should identify the specific target response you are expecting from the learner.

For instance, if a parent intends for a child to learn how to eat with a fork and spoon, then eating with a fork and spoon is the target behavior.

(32) (B) A description of circumstance under which conduct takes place, description of desired behavior, description of requirements for success.

A detailed description of the behavior makes it easy to manage a treatment program and describes the reaction that leads to positive reinforcement.

An accurately defined behavior must have three essentials: a description of the circumstance under which conduct will occur, a description of desired behavior (the goal) and a description of the requirements for success.

(33) (C) Activities that assist students in achieving their learning objectives.

An important component of skill acquisition is a learning strategy. Learning strategies are activities that help students achieve their learning objectives. These activities help obtain the result, whether teacher- or learner-centered. The learner's desired learning style greatly influences the learning strategy.

(34) (C) Teach, learn and review.

For defining an action, analysts write learning techniques using terms like *teach*, *learn*, *review*, *identify*, *perform*, *describe*, *construct* and *apply*.

(35) (D) Task analysis.

Task analysis is a crucial teaching precept to support the learner's development from fundamental to advanced skill acquisition. After skill steps are defined, the students learn them through a structured sequence of activities. These activities include multiple actions, suction reinforcement and prompting.

(36) (B) Contingent reinforcement.

Contingent reinforcement is the use of reinforcers depending on a specific behavior. Analysts consider this method the basis of ABA because it allows RBTs to reinforcc a particular behavior.

In contingent reinforcement, the individual receives the reward after completing a task. For example, students must complete all their homework problems to receive free lunch. The technique avoids reinforcing undesirable behaviors.

(37) (A) Orally, through modeling or physically.

A stimulus that helps subjects generate the reaction is known as a cue. Response cues can be administered orally, through modeling or physically.

(38) (B) Conditioned reinforcement.

Conditioned reinforcement is improved by using another reinforcer, such as awards, tokens, praise, toys or money. In contrast, unconditioned reinforcement does not need training and conditioning. Examples of unconditioned reinforcers are physical attention, painkiller, drink and food.

Intermittent reinforcement plans produce reinforcement only when particular instances of the behavior occur, as compared to continuous reinforcement schedules, which offer reinforcement for every occurrence of a behavior.

(39) (A) Positive reinforcement.

Positive reinforcement refers to a consequence being added as a result of an action. An example is a child given a favorite toy after completing a task. In this case, giving a toy is a consequence of the effort to complete the task. Positive reinforcements are not merely rewards; they only mean that action has reinforced a particular behavior.

Many of us utilize components of positive reinforcement without even realizing it. Parents use it with their children to encourage them to perform chores; teachers use it with their students to promote homework and employers use it to increase productivity.

Positive reinforcement can have five different schedules: continuous schedules, fixed ratios, fixed intervals, variable ratios and variable intervals. The reinforcement must be given immediately after the desired behavior has taken place.

Delayed reinforcement is most likely to increase the behavior. An example is a child who has earned a reward from his mother but receives it only after he starts crying. The parents support the child for crying, not for what he did to achieve it.

(40) (A) Negative enforcement.

While positive reinforcements are a consequence of an action, negative reinforcement means eliminating the product. A mother who removes the punishment of doing additional homework is an example of negative reinforcement.

Another example is someone who takes a shower to remove body odor. In ABA, taking a shower is negatively reinforced by eliminating the bad smell. Similarly, another example of negative reinforcement is turning off the lights at night, which encourages better sleep. This is an example of negative reinforcement, as the light is subtracted.

Negative reinforcement is not the exact opposite of positive reinforcement. Positive reinforcement rewards a client for showing desirable behavior, while negative reinforcement can provide a reward by eliminating an unwanted stimulus from the environment.

(41) (B) Fixed ratio, fixed interval, variable ratio, variable interval.

The reinforcement process improves an appropriate behavior, which is an essential step in behavior therapy. Schedules of reinforcement relate to how and when the consequence of conduct is provided.

Support that repeatedly occurs after the same number of responses is known as a fixed ratio. A fixed ratio of one (FR-1) in which the delivery of reinforcement happens after each response is similar to continuous reinforcement. Similarly, a fixed ratio of three (FR-3) would require three responses to occur before providing reinforcement.

A fixed ratio helps create a contingency between reinforcement and behavior. Under the fixed interval, the reinforcement is delivered for the first correct response following the passage of a given time limit. The response occurs at a lower rate with a fixed interval schedule than those on ratio schedules. So, reinforcement is always provided after a preset period with interval schedules.

Variable interval and ratio relate to situations where several reinforcements are essential. In variable ratios, the average number of a specified number of responses must be completed before receiving reinforcement. A variable interval reinforces a response after an average length of time has elapsed.

(42) (C) Variable ratio.

A variable ratio refers to a situation in which the amount of time before the reinforcement changes irregularly. It is a reinforcement in which a response is reinforced after an average number of responses. The frequency with which a behavior is reinforced can help evaluate the learning of the response. In the variable ratio method, rewards are provided after an unpredictable number of responses. There is no guarantee when a reward will be received.

However, because individuals do not know when the reward will begin, they will continue to respond each time in the hope they will receive it. For example, on average, every five bites of cauliflower result in a bite of burger. The reinforced response is a bite of burger, which happens after every five bites of cauliflower on average.

A variable ratio can be used in the classroom to help students learn efficiently. Since students do not know when they will be rewarded for completing their homework, they may be motivated to turn in all the required assignments. Slot machines are another example of a variable ratio since players do not know how many times they must play before they win.

Section 4: Behavior Reduction

(43) (B) Escape, sensory, tangibles and attention.

There are four functions of behavior. These aid in the identification of why people react the way they do. Functions of behavior include escape, sensory stimulation, access to tangibles and attention.

(44) (C) Escapist behavior.

In a situation that does not feel good or comforting, a client might choose alternatives. Escapist behavior allows clients to run away from tasks and avoid interaction.

(45) (D) Both (A) and (C).

Behavior cannot be measured simply as something requiring extra observation. It is necessary to analyze feelings and emotions to understand what the client is going through or trying to express.

However, when this is not possible, certain actions are shown in front of the RBT (real-time observation) to aid in the process. For example, covert behavior is shown through actions, not feelings.

(46) (C) It positively increases the future behavioral outlook.

Reinforcement allows an individual to be praised or punished. However, its effect depends on certain actions.

When behavior is reinforced, it helps RBTs understand the reason it happened and whether it should be encouraged or not.

(47) (A) They aid RBTs in timing when to transition.

When dealing with a client, it may not be easy to tell the individual when the time is up. This may also trigger anxiety and make things difficult.

Visual timers exist to solve this problem and provide a solution showing the individual how much time is left. They also ease transitions without making the transition obvious or pointing it out.

(48) (B) An easier and temporary replacement behavior.

Replacement behaviors are said to be quick and easier solutions to any problematic behaviors. They do not take the place of the problematic behaviors and are needed to control the situation at hand.

(49) (A) Encouragement of positive behavior.

Differential reinforcement serves as an aid to cater to special behaviors. Other behaviors are not paid much attention to during differential reinforcement because they are not the target at that moment.

In this type of reinforcement, behavior is encouraged if it is positive, meaning acceptable or conforming.

(50) (B) No. It can stop aggressive behaviors only by shifting to others.

Certain methods help limit or reduce the intensity of inappropriate behavior, but they cannot eliminate it. The process of neutral redirection plays the role of observation and helps RBTs control certain behaviors to an extent by shifting to a different mode of action and diverting feelings.

(51) (A) By analyzing essential behavioral functions.

The four primary functions must be analyzed before proceeding further to understand why any type of behavior occurs.

(52) (B) Scratching skin.

Sensory stimulation is an action that offers validation for someone or makes them feel good in a situation.

(53) (A) Four.

Four functions of behavior exist in ABA therapy to identify issues and provide a solution to certain types of behaviors. They also assist in the creation of behavior plans for clients.

(54) (C) Wear extra protective equipment and proceed with care.

If a technician is working with an aggressive client, it is important to have appropriate protection. The RBT must wear clothes that cover body areas likely to be exposed during the aggressive episode.

Section 5: Documentation and Reporting

(55) (B) Immediately ask the supervisor for assistance and guidance.

An RBT needs to communicate with the supervisor as soon as possible. Supervisors are there to guide and train. It is important to understand the seriousness of every case, and the most professional way to go forward with any query is to immediately ask the supervisor for assistance.

(56) (C) Helga should report the incident to her supervisor and work to avoid a similar mishap in the future, perhaps by implementing mechanical or digital data collection systems.

It is crucial for Helga to discuss her concerns quickly with her supervisor. The supervisor should understand that RBTs are human and can make errors.

(57) (C) Tell the supervisor or family right away about the client's behavior and condition.

In supervision, effective communication is crucial. However, an RBT must be able to distinguish between issues that require immediate attention and those that do not. To discuss concerns and problem areas swiftly and amicably, the RBT and the supervisor must make sure their communication abilities are both expressive and receptive.

(58) (A) Maintaining professional boundaries.

RBTs must always maintain professional boundaries. They must communicate politely and professionally. However, they might grow attached to clients. So, it is crucial to constantly keep in mind their position and the fact that they are offering a professional service.

Do not establish any connections outside of the client-professional service provider relationship. Also be sure to limit the conversation to professional subjects to avoid parallel connections or conflicts of interest, and do not go into detail about any personal matters (share no more than enough to maintain a friendly, professional manner).

Avoid giving your personal phone number to patients or caregivers if at all possible. If you know a potential client personally, it is best to steer clear of doing business with them.

(59) (C) "Hawke completed the handwashing procedure step by step on his own."

An RBT should make notes about objective observation during the session. While RBTs are permitted to offer their opinions, it is essential to carefully record the majority of the session notes.

So, an RBT must communicate using observable, concrete terms and include action verbs, such as running, punched, pointed, shook his head, etc. This offers an unbiased account of how the client's conduct functions and makes it simpler to comprehend the client's behavior and consider potential next moves.

For example, in between sessions, summarize the client's progress in as many sentences as you can. It will be feasible to accurately understand the client's environment if session notes are objective.

(60) (D) All of the above.

To improve their learning progress, RBTs who receive effective feedback from their supervisors should reflect on their own learning and learning practices. This feedback can be related to appropriate and inappropriate behavior, being in compliance with the laws, regulations or standards of proper behavior or practice.

(61) (C) Putting the notes in a file folder and locking them in a filing cabinet.

Any information pertaining to the client should be kept on file. Family members should not be given access to it. This includes any notes the RBT may have made during a session.

Only the concerned RBT should have access to any paper documents that are not saved electronically. The best way to do this is by having all the notes locked in a cabinet.

(62) (D) All of the above.

Under the direct supervision of a BCBA or BCaBA, the RBT's role in the service delivery system entails implementing measurement, evaluation, skill acquisition, behavior reduction, documenting and reporting, as well as maintaining professional conduct within the practice's limits.

(63) (A) Seven.

Records and information gathered by BCBAs and RBTs must be kept for at least seven years in addition to any other time periods specified by law.

(64) (D) Both (A) and (C).

Instead of analyzing why something happened, you should only describe what happened during real-time sessions to create objective session notes.

Other variables that could have an impact on the client should be noted as well. These include illnesses, relocation stress, medication, etc.

Section 6: Professional Conduct and Scope of Practice

(65) (A) Supervision.

Organizations can achieve better client outcomes through quality supervision and skilled RBTs.

(66) (D) Small talk.

RBTs should be respectful toward their clients and the clients' families. Whenever RBTs talk with a client's family, they should ensure not to engage in small talk.

Also, when RBTs are conversing with coworkers, small talk focusing on a client should be avoided. This is professional conduct.

(67) (A) Supervisory relationship.

The supervisor needs to maintain a supervisory relationship with the trainee. The Supervisor Curriculum Training Outline describes the relationship as "determining feasible supervision capacity based on available time and resources for several activities." These activities involve maintaining impactful services, preparing content for supervision, timely correspondence and access to places for supervision.

Supervisors need to record all documents that manage the supervisory relationship. Documentation includes work logs, background checks, papers for BCBA audits and contracts.

(68) (B) It will lead to RBTs engaging in a relationship outside their professional area.

It is essential for RBTs not to accept gifts from their clients or the clients' families. Taking gifts will lead to the RBTs engaging in a relationship outside their professional domain.

(69) (A) 1/2 of the supervision hours.

Supervisors need to complete the BCBA monthly experience and final experience forms. Supervision is preferred to be in-person but can be done online. A maximum of half of the supervision hours can be held in a group format.

(70) (D) Initiating the purpose of supervision, describing strategies and outcomes, entering a supervisory relationship with the trainee and making a structured plan.

According to the Supervisor Curriculum Training Outline, requirements for supervision include initiating the purpose of supervision, describing strategies and outcomes, entering a supervisory relationship with a trainee and making a structured plan.

A supervisor needs to state the purpose of supervision before providing optimum quality services to clients. RBT supervisors must identify strategies and outcomes, during which supervisors can discuss unprofessional behavior or unsatisfactory progress.

Supervisors must also prepare a supervisory relationship that includes maintenance of services, access to places for supervision, timely correspondence and content preparation. They need to create a structured plan containing content for supervision and evaluating the competency of an RBT.

(71) (A) It can compromise the RBT's and client's personal information.

RBTs should avoid providing clients' families with their phone numbers. The client or the client's family can reach an RBT through the office or by email.

(72) (A) Instruction, demonstration, observation and feedback.

There are usually four steps for the supervision of an RBT: instruction, demonstration, observation and feedback.

Initially, a supervisor must instruct the RBT concerning the different aspects he or she noticed. The supervisor must then demonstrate how the problem can be solved.

Following the demonstration, the supervisor can observe the RBT, keeping in mind the previous issues.

After observing for a final time, the supervisor then provides feedback to improve the RBT's performance.

(73) (A) This is allowed two years after the first service is provided to a client.

RBTs must avoid developing any personal relationships with their current and former clients. If an RBT desires to have a relationship with a former client, it is only permissible two years after the first service provided to the client.

(74) (A) Because RBTs may form an emotional bond with their client, which can impact their workflow.

To remain professional, RBTs must avoid giving services to their family, friends or relatives.

(75) (A) Supervision can be exhausting for RBTs, so their achievements need to be appreciated.

Initially, the supervisor sets goals for the RBT and later provides feedback once the RBT completes the goals. Although it improves performance, supervision is exhausting for RBTs. Therefore, supervisors need to appreciate the achievements of RBTs so they remain motivated.

(76) (B) Frequency recording.

Frequency recording is the most appropriate data collection method to measure how often a behavior, such as vocal stimming, occurs during a session. This method notes each instance of the behavior. It is efficient for behaviors that have a clear beginning and end.

(77) (A) Latency recording.

Latency recording measures the time that elapses from the presentation of a stimulus (such as an instruction) to the onset of the response. This method helps assess the client's responsiveness to given instructions. It also captures the delay before the client begins their response.

(78) (C) Momentary time sampling.

Momentary time sampling documents whether a behavior is present or absent at specific moments. This makes it more suitable for behaviors that do not require continuous observation. For instance, when a child raises their hand in class.

(79) (C) Permanent product recording.

Permanent product recording measures the outcomes or results of behavior after it has occurred without the need for direct observation during the behavior. It is ideal for behaviors that leave a tangible outcome or product, such as the completion of tasks (e.g., putting away toys).

(80) (C) Line graph.

A line graph illustrates changes and trends in behavior over time. It allows analysts to plot the data points connected with a line to show increases or decreases in the frequency of a behavior.

(81) (A) Free-operant observations.

Free-operant observations allow a client to choose activities without direct interaction pressure. Simultaneously, the RBT observes the client's choices and identifies what activities might motivate them to communicate.

(82) (B) Use a multiple stimulus with replacement assessment daily.

For clients who have various preferences, a multiple stimulus with replacement assessment records current interests and provides a variety of stimuli. The RBT can perform this assessment daily to keep engagement high.

(83) (D) Free-operant observations.

This approach minimizes aggression triggers as it allows clients to engage freely with items and prevents direct choice pressure. It is best for children prone to aggression during transitions.

(84) (A) Paired stimulus.

This method simplifies decisions for clients who struggle with multiple choices as it presents only two options at a time. It also reduces frustration and increases participation. Overall, it is ideal to identify effective reinforcers for clients overwhelmed by too many choices.

(85) (B) Introduce novel stimuli in a free-operant observation setting.

To overcome progress plateaus, an RBT should introduce new stimuli, which re-engage the client. This will revitalize motivation and aid in continuous skill development.

Test 2

Section 1: Measurement

(1) In what form of measurement procedures do you measure every instance of behavior within the entire observation period?

(A) Whole interval sampling.

(B) Continuous sampling.

(C) Momentary time sampling.

(D) Discontinuous sampling.

(2) An RBT counted every time Jim ate chalk. Jim ate chalk six times. This is an example of _____.

(A) Rate.

(B) Latency.

(C) Frequency.

(D) Baseline.

(3) An RBT uses duration recording to collect data on how long Alice can sit in her seat during a 15-minute class. Alice remained in her seat for 10 minutes.

Which of the following would the RBT enter in the session notes?

(A) 0.1.

(B) 10 minutes.

(C) 5 minutes.

(D) 2/3.

(4) Which of the following is not a type of discontinuous measurement procedure?

(A) Partial interval recording.

(B) Momentary time sampling.

(C) Primary reinforcement.

(D) Whole interval recording.

(5) Partial interval recording has a tendency __________.

(A) To underestimate the frequency of the target behavior.

(B) To be the perfect estimate of the target behavior.

(C) To overestimate the frequency of the target behavior.

(D) To overestimate the latency of the target behavior.

(6) Lucas began to brush his teeth 10 minutes after his mother told him to. This is an example of _______.

(A) Latency.

(B) Frequency.

(C) Momentary sample.

(D) Topography.

(7) Which of the following measurements refers to how long a behavior occurred?

(A) Count.

(B) Duration.

(C) Response latency.

(D) Celeration.

(8) An RBT would use ____________ interval recording when the behavior of interest occurs throughout the entire interval. This type of measurement is used when the target behavior occurs at a __________ rate.

(A) Partial; high.

(B) Partial; low.

(C) Whole; low.

(D) Whole; high.

(9) ______ means keeping track of tangible items or environmental effects (e.g., crayons thrown on the ground or completed written worksheets) caused by a particular behavior.

(A) Permanent-product recording.

(B) Momentary time sampling.

(C) Reinforcement sampling.

(D) Paired choice recording.

(10) It is crucial to _________ when entering a data point on a behavioral graph.

(A) Write down the date of the observation.

(B) Use a straight line to join the data to the previous point on the graph under the same circumstances.

(C) Note the staff member's or observer's initials.

(D) All of the above.

(11) At the two-minute mark of each observation time, an RBT checks his watch to assess if the client is actively engaged. The RBT takes another look at the two-minute, four-minute and six-minute marks.

If the client is working at the time, the RBT notes a + mark to indicate the client was engaged in the process. This measurement is known as _________.

(A) Whole interval recording.

(B) Partial interval recording.

(C) Momentary time sampling.

(D) Whole-time sampling.

(12) Which of the following is an example of measurable and observable behavior analysis?

(A) Dina is aggressive and cunning.

(B) Dina hit her sister.

(C) Dina won the game five times in 10 minutes.

(D) Dina is aggressive. So, she hit her sister.

Section 2: Assessment

(13) In which of the following preference assessments would you observe how long a client engages with an item and the items she engaged with?

(A) Multiple stimulus without replacement preference assessments.

(B) Free-operant observation preference assessments.

(C) Multiple stimulus with replacement preference assessments.

(D) Paired-stimulus preference assessments.

(14) The assessment of curriculum-based, developmental and social skills, typically in the form of an interview or a check-off list of activities, is known as __________.

(A) Individualized assessment.

(B) Functional assessment.

(C) Paired stimulus.

(D) Direct assessment.

(15) An RBT provides her client with an array of six items and records which item the client chooses. The chosen item is removed from the collection, the remaining items' order or replacement is rearranged and the next trial begins with fewer items in the array.

Again, the RBT records the item the client chooses from the array. This kind of assessment is known as ______.

(A) Preference assessment.

(B) Free operant assessment.

(C) Functional assessment.

(D) ABC recording.

(16) A stimulus preference assessment is conducted _______________ the reinforcer assessment.

(A) Before.

(B) After.

(C) Simultaneously with.

(D) As a substitute of.

(17) Which of the following is not a typical function of behavior?

(A) Antecedent.

(B) Automatic reinforcement.

(C) Escape.

(D) Attention seeking.

(18) What are two kinds of indirect functional behavior assessments?

(A) Behavioral interviews and behavior rating scales.

(B) Functional and central analysis.

(C) Contingent escape.

(D) Descriptive functional behavior and multiple-stimulus preference assessments.

Section 3: Skill Acquisition

(19) Which of the following contains discrete-trial teaching sections?

(A) Instructions, the learner's response and the reinforcer.

(B) Instructions, teaching skills and the reinforcer.

(C) Instructions, the reinforcer and matching objects.

(D) Instructions, the learner's response and functions.

(20) Which of the following best describes treatment and education procedures for teaching skills to ASD learners?

(A) Reinforcement.

(B) Discrete-trial teaching.

(C) Instruction.

(D) Motor and vocal imitation.

(21) What are the four essential components of DTT?

(A) Discriminative stimulus, the prompt, client's response and consequence and the inter-trial period.

(B) Discriminative stimulus, the reinforcer, client's response and consequence, inter-trial period.

(C) Discriminative stimulus, the prompt, client's response and discrete-trial teaching.

(D) The prompt, client's response, consequence and inter-trial period.

(22) What is the most suitable component of DDT to help a client come up with the correct response?

(A) Discriminative stimulus.

(B) Inter-trial period.

(C) Discrete-trial teaching.

(D) The prompt.

(23) Which of the following features the steps of conducting DTT?

(A) Initiate the inter-trial period, wait for a correct response, immediately record data and regain the learner's attention while presenting the next instruction.

(B) Deliver the instruction, wait for a correct response, immediately record data and regain the learner's attention while presenting the next instruction.

(C) Deliver the instruction, wait 10 seconds for the correct response, immediately record data and regain the learner's attention while presenting the next instruction.

(D) Deliver the instruction, wait three seconds for the learner to respond, immediately record data and regain the learner's attention while presenting the next instruction.

(24) A behavior analyst wants to use a strategy that employs applied behavior analysis principles to provide organized learning opportunities by leveraging the learner's natural interests and motivation.

What is this strategy called?

(A) General teaching.

(B) Behavioral teaching.

(C) Incidental teaching.

(D) Positive reinforcement.

(25) John is a child with poor language skills. During a lesson, Derek, a preschool teacher, places a toy out of John's reach. John notices the toy and asks Derek to bring it closer, starting communication with Derek. Derek compliments John and hands him the toy.

What is the response and reinforcement in this incident?

(A) There is no response or reinforcement.

(B) They cannot be determined.

(C) The response is John communicating with Derek, and the reinforcement is Derek complimenting John and handing him the toy.

(D) The reinforcement is John communicating with Derek, and the response is Derek complimenting John and handing him the toy.

(26) Derek is training another student in his class, Abraham, who loves the color yellow. He put a bright yellow pencil out of Abraham's reach. Abraham shows delayed communication by failing to request the pencil.

Derek points at Abraham and explains that he has no idea what Abraham wants. Abraham points to the pencil, and Derek hands him the pencil as a reward.

What is the prompt and the reinforcement in this situation?

(A) The prompt is when Derek points at Abraham and explains he has no idea what Abraham wants, and the reinforcement is when Derek hands the pencil to Abraham as a reward.

(B) The reinforcement is Abraham has no idea what he wants, and the prompt is when Derek gives the pencil to Abraham as a reward.

(C) There is no response or reinforcement.

(D) They cannot be determined.

(27) Why is the learner's current interest determined in the natural environment?

(A) To increase engagement.

(B) To evaluate a successful response.

(C) To have a face-to-face interaction.

(D) To control the environment.

(28) A trainer arranges a play area for a learner where toys are stored in containers and categorized by category.

What is the environment?

(A) Toys.

(B) Play area.

(C) Containers.

(D) Trainer.

(29) What can the trainer use to encourage the learner to reply?

(A) Reinforcement.

(B) Environment.

(C) Nonverbal cues.

(D) Attention.

(30) Which of the following best describes repetitive reinforcement for a learner?

(A) Several chances to practice a newly obtained skill.

(B) One chance to practice newly obtained skills.

(C) External conditions to help obtain new skills.

(D) No chances to practice a newly obtained skill.

(31) A behavior intervention that connects a series of behaviors creates a more complex behavior chain that is called _________.

(A) Repetitive reinforcement.

(B) Behavior formation.

(C) Behavior analysis.

(D) Task analysis.

(32) Which of the following contains several behavior chains of task analysis?

(A) Forward chaining, backward chaining, backward chaining with a leap ahead and total task chaining.

(B) Forward chaining, general chaining, backward chaining with a leap ahead and total task chaining.

(C) Forward chaining, repetitive chaining, backward chaining with a leap ahead and total task chaining.

(D) General chaining, backward chaining, backward chaining with a leap ahead and total task chaining.

(33) Which of the following best describes reinforcement backed through the chain and reinforcing the end of the sequence?

(A) Forward chaining.

(B) Backward chaining.

(C) Backward chaining with a leap ahead.

(D) Total task chaining.

(34) Which of the following terms refers to a learner's ability to understand differences between two or more things?

(A) Discrimination training.

(B) Total task changing.

(C) Behavioral training.

(D) Random rotation.

(35) The entire sequence is completed, and reinforcement is received at the end of the task chain.

What type of behavior chain is this?

(A) Forward chaining.

(B) Backward chaining.

(C) Backward chaining with a leap ahead.

(D) Total task chaining.

(36) Which of the following behavior chains begins with assistance with all the steps except the last?

(A) Forward chaining.

(B) Backward chaining.

(C) Backward chaining with a leap ahead.

(D) Total task chaining.

(37) A behavior chain includes the leap-ahead procedure, which reduces the training time required to learn the chain.

Which behavior chain is this?

(A) Forward chaining.

(B) Backward chaining.

(C) Backward chaining with a leap ahead.

(D) Total task chaining.

(38) Two or more stimuli are implemented and alternated. The RBT asks about each stimulus at random.

What is this method called?

(A) Discrimination.

(B) Mass trials.

(C) Behavioral training.

(D) Random rotation.

(39) ________ allows learners to differentiate between two or more stimuli simultaneously.

(A) General discrimination.

(B) Simultaneous discrimination.

(C) Behavioral discrimination.

(D) Random rotation.

(40) Which of the following includes the different ways simultaneous discrimination is conducted?

(A) Mass trials, random rotation and general rotation.

(B) Mass trials, mass trials with a distractor and random rotation.

(C) General trials, mass rotation and random rotation.

(D) Mass trials, mass trials with a distractor and general rotation.

(41) What is a procedure in which you present trials on a repeated basis of the same simple discrimination?

(A) A mass trial.

(B) A mass trial with a distractor.

(C) A random rotation.

(D) Successive discrimination.

(42) "We do one thing in the presence of one stimulus and then do something else later in the presence of another."

What does the above sentence describe?

(A) Mass trials.

(B) Mass trial with a distractor.

(C) Random rotation.

(D) Successive discrimination.

Section 4: Behavior Reduction

(43) Adam slaps his little brother, Jamie. His father makes Adam face the wall for 20 minutes. When Adam comes back, he hits Jamie again. Adam's father tells him to face the wall again.

Adam's father's action is an example of ________.

(A) Positive reinforcement.

(B) Extinction.

(C) Negative reinforcement.

(D) Positive punishment.

(44) What happens during an extinction burst?

(A) Negative behavior is increased.

(B) Behavior turns positive.

(C) Redirection occurs.

(D) The situation does not change.

(45) What is the most effective method to help a client decide what to do?

(A) Talking loudly.

(B) Forcing the client to choose.

(C) Using images or objects.

(D) Giving rewards.

(46) Which of the following is a coping strategy?

(A) Screaming, throwing items and arguing.

(B) Distracting with objects and breathing to calm down.

(C) Counting loudly.

(D) None of the above.

(47) What is the primary goal of using functional communication?

(A) Describing issues.

(B) Engaging coping strategies.

(C) Displaying negative reinforcement.

(D) Assisting with a replacement behavior.

(48) How is the process of extinction defined in ABA?

(A) Encouraging all types of behavior.

(B) Withdrawing reinforcement to discourage negative behavior.

(C) Inducing change through punishment.

(D) Both (A) and (B).

(49) How can professional technicians deal with aggressive behaviors?

(A) By walking away from the situation for a while.

(B) By rewarding the individual.

(C) By carefully assessing the situation or moving away.

(D) By talking loudly and making the other person understand that what he or she is doing is wrong.

(50) What is an example of access to tangibles?

(A) A child screaming when he wants ice cream.

(B) A child playing with toys.

(C) A child crying due to an injury.

(D) A mother rewarding a child.

(51) What does a functional behavior assessment do?

(A) It plays no significant role and is a formality.

(B) It entertains the client.

(C) It helps the technician choose a client.

(D) It helps the RBT identify why particular behavior occurs.

(52) What can be done to help some children with ASD transition?

(A) Encourage and offer rewards.

(B) Move away from the situation.

(C) Use different methods and observe their feelings.

(D) Constantly change their environments.

(53) Why is some behavior not seen?

(A) Because it is covert or appears in the form of feelings.

(B) Because the client takes no action.

(C) Because it is not present.

(D) Because of inaccurate and invalid observation.

(54) Which of the following could be an example of escapist behavior?

(A) A child playing cheerfully.

(B) A teenager running away from home.

(C) Eating loudly.

(D) A mom punishing her children.

Section 5: Documentation and Reporting

(55) Your supervisor instructs you to employ a technique you are unfamiliar with. What should you do in this situation?

(A) Pretend to know what the supervisor is talking about and after the session is over, look it up on the internet.

(B) Become irritated at the supervisor for not knowing what you've been trained to do.

(C) Apologize for not knowing how to use the strategy and offer to look it up later on the internet.

(D) Admit to the supervisor immediately that you do not know how to use the strategy and ask to be shown how to do it.

(56) RBTs support service delivery while being carefully monitored and directed by ________.

(A) A BCBA who is also an RBT supervisor.

(B) A skilled RBT and an RBT supervisor.

(C) An RBT requirements coordinator or supervisor.

(D) An ACE coordinator or RBT supervisor.

(57) Which of the following best describes documentation in the context of an RBT's job?

(A) Data collection.

(B) Incidents recording.

(C) Generating objective session notes.

(D) All of the above.

(58) An RBT utilizes a spreadsheet program and computer to graph data. Which of the following is the best technique to guarantee the confidentiality of the information?

(A) Take a printout because you should not leave any electronic footprint.

(B) Protect the passwords used to access the computer and spreadsheet program.

(C) Leave the program as it is; no one can read the complicated data.

(D) Upload the data to a cloud network utilized by the client's family and delete it from your computer.

(59) Never doing or saying anything to cause embarrassment to the client is a part of maintaining ________.

(A) Professional boundaries.

(B) The client's dignity.

(C) The ABC method.

(D) Closeness with the client.

(60) Which of the following is not a part of the professional and ethical compliance code?

(A) Accuracy and data use.

(B) Maintaining confidentiality.

(C) Documentation of professional work and research.

(D) Marketing the agency.

(61) You and your client are set to begin your session. What should you do to ensure you are prepared for a successful session?

(A) You can wing it. After all, you are excellent at this and your memory is phenomenal.

(B) Everyone only requires a cup of coffee; if they claim otherwise, they are either misrepresenting their needs or tea drinkers.

(C) You should be familiar with the functions and definitions of the response you will be gauging during your session. Additionally, ensure you have everything you will need to collect data, including pens, paper and pencils.

(D) You should conduct functional behavioral and informal preference assessments before the session. Make a therapy plan after that as well.

(62) Which steps should you take if you learn that a client's legal rights are being violated?

(A) Speak with your supervisor.

(B) Observe the company's policies.

(C) Call the authorities.

(D) All of the above.

(63) All except which of the following are appropriate methods of responding to feedback from your supervisor?

(A) Justifying your actions because the supervisor could be mistaken in his or her feedback.

(B) Attempting to improve services.

(C) Implementing the feedback.

(D) None of the above.

(64) At least what percent of an RBT's total direct hours worked each month must be supervised?

(A) 2.

(B) 5.

(C) 10.

(D) 20.

Section 6: Professional Conduct and Scope of Practice

(65) An RBT has personal issues with smoking and observes one of her client's family members smoking.

How should the RBT deal with this client?

(A) The RBT should interact with this client the same way she does with others.

(B) The RBT should not work with this client.

(C) The RBT is not allowed to work with this client.

(D) The RBT should differentiate between this client and others.

(66) Is it ethical for an RBT to have random conversations with coworkers about clients?

(A) Yes, but only if the coworker is aware of the client.

(B) It is not ethical under any circumstances.

(C) It is allowed under some circumstances.

(D) It is ethical under all circumstances.

(67) If an RBT becomes aware that false information was given to the BCBA, the RBT must ________.

(A) Instantly inform the BCBA.

(B) Ignore the false information.

(C) Avoid informing the BCBA.

(D) None of the above.

(68) An RBT becomes aware of the possibility that certain events need to be self-reported.
How long does the RBT have to complete the self-reporting process?

(A) 120 days.

(B) 90 days.

(C) 60 days.

(D) 30 days.

(69) Based on the Supervisor Curriculum Training Outline, people who supervise RBTs must complete training for ___ hours.

(A) Eight.

(B) Six.

(C) Four.

(D) Two.

(70) In the latest session, a client misbehaves with Derek, an RBT.

What should Derek do?

(A) He should make aggressive remarks.

(B) He should retaliate.

(C) He should ignore the misbehavior.

(D) He should notify his supervisor and concerned authorities.

(71) When can RBTs share their clients' information with their supervisors?

(A) RBTs are not allowed to share information under any circumstance.

(B) RBTs can share their clients' information at any time.

(C) RBTs can share their clients' information only after gaining consent.

(D) RBTs cannot share information even if they acquire the clients' consent.

(72) Is it permissible for an RBT to discuss a client's information with family members?

(A) RBTs should not discuss client-specific information with family.

(B) RBTs are allowed to discuss information about clients with the client's family members.

(C) RBTs can discuss information by gaining the supervisor's consent.

(D) None of the above.

(73) John is an RBT who shares his social media platform links with his clients. He also follows his clients on social media.

Which of the following is true about John's behavior?

(A) It is unprofessional because it will create a bond between John and his clients.

(B) It is professional.

(C) It may or may not be professional; the verdict lies with the clients.

(D) It depends on the supervisor's policy.

(74) Why should an RBT avoid giving unnecessary advice to stakeholders?

(A) It is against the law.

(B) It is against the supervisor's policy.

(C) It could lead to accidents that jeopardize the client's safety.

(D) It shows a lack of professionalism.

(75) What must RBTs remember before any conversation with stakeholders?

(A) They can start any conversation without the client's consent.

(B) They are responsible for promising results to stakeholders.

(C) They should give unnecessary advice.

(D) They need to acquire consent before proceeding with the session.

(76) An RBT works with a nine-year-old boy who has ASD to improve his social interaction skills. The boy shows interest in various topics but struggles to start discussions. Which reinforcement strategy should the RBT prioritize to encourage the boy to initiate conversations?

(A) Provide verbal praise every time the boy initiates a conversation.

(B) Use a token economy system.

(C) Provide a preferred toy or activity after every attempt.

(D) Ignore unsuccessful attempts.

(77) A behavior analyst designs a skill acquisition plan for a fifteen-year-old girl with intellectual disability to teach her money management skills. Which of the following should be the first step in her skill acquisition plan?

(A) Establish a baseline of her current money management skills.

(B) Implement a token economy to reinforce correct money management.

(C) Use discrete trial education to introduce concepts of money.

(D) Introduce a variety of money-related apps to enhance learning.

(78) During a session with a seven-year-old child with ASD, an RBT is tasked to teach him how to tie his shoes. The supervisor recommends that they break down the task into smaller steps. What is the name of this approach?

(A) Task analysis.

(B) Forward chaining.

(C) Total task chaining.

(D) Backward chaining.

(79) A teenager with ADHD learns new organizational skills to manage his schoolwork more effectively. The behavior analyst has noticed that the teenager responds well to visual cues. Which strategy would be most effective to support this skill acquisition?

(A) Use verbal instructions to guide task completion.

(B) Create a visual schedule and checklist for daily and weekly tasks.

(C) Implement a reward system for every task completed without visual aids.

(D) Focus on naturalistic teaching methods without the use of visual supports.

(80) An RBT uses discrete trial teaching (DTT) to help a four-year-old girl with ASD increase her vocabulary. The girl is highly motivated by social stories and interactive play. How should the RBT incorporate these interests into the DTT sessions?

(A) Integrate social stories and interactive play as part of the consequences for correct responses.

(B) Use social stories and interactive play at the end of the session.

(C) Avoid the use of social stories and interactive play to keep the session structured.

(D) Focus exclusively on verbal praise as reinforcement.

(81) A seven-year-old with ASD hits peers to escape group tasks. What replacement behavior should the team teach?

(A) Use communication cards to request a break.

(B) Prohibit participation.

(C) Engage in a different activity without permission.

(D) Wait for the activity to end without interaction.

(82) A ten-year-old screams for attention in class. Which differential reinforcement strategy is best?

(A) Reinforce any quiet behavior.

(B) Ignore all screams.

(C) Reward the child when they raise their hand to speak.

(D) Give a timeout for screaming.

(83) A child flaps their hands when anxious. Which extinction method addresses this sensory behavior?

(A) Remove the anxiety-provoking stimulus.

(B) Ignore the hand-flapping.

(C) Provide a stress ball as an alternative.

(D) Teach deep breaths.

(84) A student leaves their seat frequently during lessons. Which strategy could effectively reduce this behavior?

(A) Apply a visual timer to signal seated periods.

(B) Reward the students who remain seated.

(C) Increase the frequency of physical activity breaks.

(D) Assign extra work each time the student leaves their seat.

(85) A child grabs toys from others without their permission. What replacement behavior should be encouraged?

(A) Ask peers for a turn with the toy.

(B) Play alone to avoid the need to share.

(C) Watch others play without participation.

(D) Retrieve a teacher to intervene each time.

Test 2: Answers and Explanations

Section 1: Measurement

(1) (B) Continuous sampling.

A continuous sampling measurement observes every instance of behavior that occurs during a class, session or day. In contrast, discontinuous measurement procedures record only a sample of behavior.

Moreover, a discontinuous sampling measurement is typically reserved for situations where resources, time or data on multiple students are limited. However, as an RBT, you will primarily use continuous measurement.

(2) (C) Frequency.

Frequency is the number of times a behavior or act is performed. It is a count or tally. So, in this case, six is the frequency of Jim eating chalk.

Rate is defined as frequency divided by time, and latency is a measurement of time between the instruction (prompt) and the beginning of response (SD).

(3) (B) 10 minutes.

Data is a calculation of how long a behavior occurs. If you want to find out how long a client takes to complete a task, start the timer when the client begins the activity and stop it when the client completes it. The time elapsed between the starting and ending points is the duration.

In the example, Alice was assigned the task of sitting in a chair during a 15-minute class. She sat for 10 minutes. So, her task duration was 10 minutes. Thus, the RBT will enter the duration in the session notes.

(4) (C) Primary reinforcement.

Discontinuous measurement types include partial interval, whole interval and momentary time sampling.

Biologically necessary stimuli for an organism, such as food, water, sleep, shelter and safety, are called primary reinforcers. They lead to involuntary responses, such as drooling when you are hungry and shown food.

(5) (A) To underestimate the frequency of the target behavior.

Partial interval recording keeps track of whether or not behavior occurred during an interval. However, it often overestimates the behavior's duration and underestimates high-frequency behaviors.

(6) (A) Latency.

Latency is a measurement of time between the prompt and the SD. In this case, the mother telling Lucas to brush his teeth is a prompt. Lucas brushing his teeth is the response. Ten minutes is the latency.

(7) (B) Duration.

Duration is a measurement of how long a behavior occurred. The number of occurrences of behavior is referred to as its count or frequency, while celeration describes how the rate of response changes over time.

Response latency is the time that elapses between the occurrence of the SD and the onset of the behavior.

(8) (D) Whole; high.

Whole interval recording is used for behaviors that do not have a clear beginning or ending or behaviors that occur at high rates.

RBTs use whole interval recording to check if the behavior continues without interruption during the given interval. They may count the number of intervals in which the behavior occurred throughout the interval.

(9) (A) Permanent-product recording.

The permanent-product recording method entails selecting a product or result that demonstrates the occurrence of the target or replacement behavior.

In this method, you record whether or not a product is produced. Some examples include homework, scratches on the body, etc.

(10) (D) All of the above.

It is important to record all information when entering a data point on a behavioral graph. This includes noting down the date of the observation and the staff member's or observer's initials. A straight line should be used to join the data to the previous point on the graph.

(11) (C) Momentary time sampling.

A sample of the defined behavior at the precise moment that data is being collected is known as momentary time sampling. The RBT would set a time mark, two minutes in this case and record at the end of the time mark. The RBT would then record whether the behavior was occurring or absent at the two-minute mark.

(12) (C) Dina won the game five times in 10 minutes.

A technician must present measurable data, such as a frequency or rate, rather than a judgment.

In the question, the observation "Dina is aggressive or cunning" is a conclusion. However, Dina winning the game five times in 10 minutes is a measurable and observable behavior that may suggest that Dina is good at the game.

Section 2: Assessment

(13) (B) Free-operant observation preference assessments.

The timing and observation of how long clients interact with an item and which items they interact with are known as free operant observation. The free-operant observation approach allows RBTs to understand that the longer clients spend on a particular activity, the more they prefer that activity.

In comparison, during multiple stimuli without replacement preference assessments, RBTs provide clients with an array of items (often toys or sweets) and ask them to choose one. RBTs take the item out of the collection after the clients use it or consume it. They note the array's items and the clients' choice of items in the array's order.

In the multiple stimuli with replacement preference assessment, RBTs present the clients with various items (usually toys or edibles) and allow them to choose one. After the clients use or consume the item, RBTs replace it in the array and substitute the unselected items with new ones.

In paired-stimulus preference assessments, stimuli are presented in pairs until every other stimulus has been presented with one another. Then the hierarchy of preferences is generated.

(14) (A) Individualized assessment.

In an individualized assessment, the RBT can conduct interviews with the client, collect baseline data by observing the client's behaviors in the individual's natural environment or probe the client by asking him or her to perform a task without assistance.

An individualized assessment gathers information about the client to determine what the client currently knows and what his or her needs are.

(15) (A) Preference assessment.

The question is specifically talking about multiple stimulus without replacement preference assessments. In this assessment, the items put in an array are identified by the RBT. Although there is no predetermined number, a reasonable collection contains roughly six to eight items.

An RBT presents a client with an array of items (often toys or sweets) and asks the person to choose one. The RBT then takes the item out of the collection after the client uses it or consumes it. Again, the RBT checks which item was preferred by the client from the remaining array. Then the RBT lists the items in a hierarchical sequence.

(16) (A) Before.

A preference assessment is conducted before the reinforcement assessment. There is a clear distinction between reinforcer and preference assessments, even though both aim to identify efficient reinforcers.

While reinforcer assessments evaluate the effectiveness of potential reinforcers, preference assessments determine the possible reinforcers. You employ preference assessments before putting reinforcement into action.

The reinforcer assessment is carried out using the data gathered about the reinforcer's impact during implementation.

(17) (A) Antecedent.

The typical functions of behavior include escape, attention seeking, automatic reinforcement and seeking access to certain things. This means that people behave in a certain way to ensure they get specific results.

The antecedent is not a function of behavior. It is an event that occurs before a behavior.

(18) (A) Behavioral interviews and behavior rating scales.

Rating scales, questionnaires and interviews are examples of indirect functional approaches. The objective is to acquire data to examine the cause of a client's behavior with the help of the client's guardians or support group.

In contrast, function analysis is a direct method of functional assessment. It is conducted by testing various conditions and contrived scenarios. An escape contingency occurs when a specific behavior disrupts an ongoing event.

A descriptive functional behavior assessment allows RBTs to observe the problem behavior in the client's natural environment.

Section 3: Skill Acquisition

(19) (A) Instructions, the learner's response and the reinforcer.

Discrete-trial teaching is one of the most recognized treatment and education procedures for teaching skills to ASD learners. It is a technique in which learning trials are done in succession, with each trial having a clear start and end.

There are three sections in DTT: the instruction, the learner's response and the reinforcer. RBTs break the skills down into small sections and provide instructions as clearly as possible. They teach each section until students master it.

In the last section, incentives reinforce learning. The point at which the trainer offers the incentives must be consistent.

(20) (B) Discrete-trial teaching.

Discrete-trial training helps autistic children learn new skills. These skills range from fundamental to complex and depend on a child's specific needs.

DTT can help autistic children learn daily living skills like writing, dressing, following instructions, etc. The training is based on the idea that you can teach any skill by breaking it into smaller steps.

Step-by-step instructions make the skills easier to learn. DTT uses repetition, so children have several opportunities to learn and adopt new skills. It also uses rewards to encourage children to acquire new skills.

(21) (A) Discriminative stimulus, the prompt, client's response and consequence and the inter-trial period.

The essential components of DTT include the discriminative stimulus, the prompt, the client's response and the consequence and the inter-trial period. A discriminative stimulus is a brief instruction that alerts the client to work. It helps the client connect a specific direction to a suitable response.

The prompt is needed to help the client come up with an accurate answer. The RBT conducts the prompt between the response and discriminative stimulus. The client's response to a stimulus may be correct or incorrect.

The last stage of DTT is the inter-trial period. It follows the outcome and leads to the conclusion of one trial while signaling the beginning of another.

(22) (D) The prompt.

The prompt is required to help the client develop the correct response. RBTs can use several types of prompts as teaching aids.

An example is a student who is learning to point to colored cards. The teacher can provide the prompt, "Point to the yellow card," and a student should then point to the yellow card. If the student responds accurately by pointing to the yellow card, the teacher can deliver a reinforcement.

No prompting is equivalent to independent. Independent prompt levels allow teachers to understand they should not use any prompts because children can respond on their own.

(23) (D) Deliver the instruction, wait three seconds for the learner to respond, immediately record data and regain the learner's attention while presenting the next instruction.

Discrete-trial teaching has four steps: delivering the instruction, waiting three seconds for the learner to respond, quickly recording data and regaining the learner's attention while presenting the next instruction.

The technician can deliver the instructions in a session. For instance, he can say, "Put your hands behind your back." The RBT should pair a prompt with the instruction if it is a prompted trail. He should also put his hands behind his back to help the client.

After giving the instructions, the RBT should wait three seconds for the learner to respond. If the learner does not respond correctly, the technician should repeat the instruction while providing a quick prompt.

When the learner responds correctly, the technician should quickly record the data. He should regain the learner's attention by giving the next instruction.

(24) (C) Incidental teaching.

Incidental training is a technique that uses ABA principles to give organized learning opportunities. It provides opportunities in a natural environment by leveraging the learner's natural interest. This training involves a skill that does not have a beginning or an end.

Incidental training is effective for a skill that someone acquires naturally over time. It is particularly beneficial for young children because it does not require direct instruction.

(25) (C) The response is John communicating with Derek, and the reinforcement is Derek complimenting John and handing him the toy.

A response is a single and specific instance of a behavior. When John notices the toy, he initiates communication with Derek and asks him to bring the toy closer. Communication is a response since John closes the distance between the toy and himself. When Derek compliments John and hands him the toy, it acts as a reinforcement to support his behavior.

A reinforcer is anything that the client may enjoy, such as toys, candy, praise, etc. Following the behavior, the reinforcer increases the probability of the behavior happening again. So, reinforcement will encourage John to perform the same behavior again.

(26) (A) The prompt is when Derek points at Abraham and explains he has no idea what Abraham wants, and the reinforcement is when Derek hands the pencil to Abraham as a reward.

Prompting refers to encouraging the use of a particular skill. It enables clients to perform a task until they learn how to do it independently. Derek's confusion works as a prompt in this scenario.

Reinforcement increases the likelihood of a behavior happening again. When Derek hands the pencil to Abraham as a reward, it acts as a reinforcement and the pencil acts as a reward, increasing the chances of Abraham performing the same behavior again.

(27) (A) To increase engagement.

A learner's current interest is determined to increase engagement. You can note which actions, objects or materials motivate the learner at any time.

However, a client's interest can change over time. For instance, if a child learner is playing with a toy car and a trainer wants to work on color identification, the RBT should not replace the toy with flash cards the child had earlier shown interest in. Instead, using the toy car in the session will increase engagement.

(28) (B) Play area.

When a trainer arranges a play area for learners, the environment is the play area itself.

(29) (C) Nonverbal cues.

RBTs can ask learners to reply by using nonverbal cues like a questioning expression, puzzled body language and an expectant gaze. They can provide more prompts for the appropriate reaction if nonverbal clues are insufficient.

(30) (A) Several chances to practice a newly obtained skill.

Repetitive reinforcement means giving a learner several chances to correct behavior. It does not limit the learner and allows the individual to gain confidence in their abilities.

(31) (D) Task analysis.

A behavior intervention that connects several or a series of behaviors to form a more complex behavior chain is known as task analysis. It breaks complex tasks down into a sequence of smaller or simpler actions and teaches clients how to perform tasks, such as completing work, eating, playing, etc.

Task analysis is helpful in desensitization programs, such as helping individuals tolerate haircuts, buzzer sounds or tooth brushing. An RBT can validate the task analysis by observing a person carry out an action sequence or consulting an expert about the tasks to be taught.

(32) (A) Forward chaining, backward chaining, backward chaining with a leap ahead and total task chaining.

There are four task analysis chaining methods: forward chaining, backward chaining, backward chaining with a leap ahead and total task chaining.

(33) (C) Backward chaining with a leap ahead.

Backward chaining with a leap ahead describes reinforcement that is backed through the chain until the student leaps ahead and is reinforced by the RBT.

(34) (A) Discrimination training.

Discrimination training refers to the learner's ability to comprehend the differences between two or more things. During training, RBTs often refer to different language operands, such as the mand, interverbal, etc.

This type of training aims to teach the child to differentiate between names and labels when asked.

(35) (D) Total task chaining.

Total task chaining means completing a sequence and receiving reinforcement at the end of the task chain. It is suitable when the learner has prerequisite skills to complete tasks in the chain and does not require several trials to criterion based on previous knowledge.

For instance, it was difficult for a child to turn on a tap and get soap, but he could do other steps the RBT had taught using prompts. For a child with autism, this type of behavior chain may be too complicated. So, RBTs prefer backward or forward chaining for children with autism.

(36) (B) Backward chaining.

Backward chaining begins with assistance with all the steps except for the last. The RBT and the child go through each step together until they reach the final step, where the RBT prompts the child to complete the process by himself or herself.

After that, both the child and the RBT move back through stages until the child learns the entire process.

(37) (C) Backward chaining with a leap ahead.

Backward chaining with a leap ahead is similar to backward chaining. Steps can be skipped, and the leap-forward procedure decreases the training time required to learn the chain.

The RBT must complete the steps in the correct order to provide proper reinforcement to the client.

(38) (D) Random rotation.

Random rotation concerns using two or more stimuli and alternating between asking for each at random.

(39) (B) Simultaneous discrimination.

Simultaneous discrimination allows learners to differentiate between two or more stimuli simultaneously. The RBT can conduct simultaneous discrimination in different ways, including mass trials with a distractor and random rotation.

(40) (B) Mass trials, mass trials with a distractor and random rotation.

Mass trials are procedures in which you repeatedly present trials of simple discrimination. An example is placing a toy on the table and giving the instruction: “Touch the toy.” The learner has to respond by touching the toy. The trial is repeated twice, with the most accurate response reinforced.

A mass trial with a distractor is a mass trial with another stimulus. For instance, you can place two toys on the table and ask the learner to touch one specific toy while changing the position of the toys frequently.

The third type of discrimination is random rotation. It involves putting together two or more stimuli and alternating between asking for each at random.

(41) (A) A mass trial.

Mass trials are procedures in which you repeatedly present trials of simple discrimination.

(42) (D) Successive discrimination.

Successive discrimination occurs when we do one thing in the presence of one stimulus and then do something else in the presence of another.

For instance, if you say, “Tell me about something that moves,” the subsequent trial will say, “Tell me about something that flies.”

Section 4: Behavior Reduction

(43) (C) Negative reinforcement.

The father’s action is an example of negative reinforcement. Over time, Adam will learn not to commit the unpleasant action because he will face similar consequences.

(44) (A) Negative behavior is increased.

During an extinction burst, there is a significant increase in unwanted behavior. It does not affect the entire teaching process and decreases on its own.

(45) (C) Using images or objects.

Showing children visuals has been found to increase the probability of them following their parents and obeying rules. Visuals also increase children's decision-making ability, allowing easier transition to new tasks.

RBTs use visual objects or photos to help learners understand the task for transition. If a learner is allowed to create a schedule and know what to do, this will make things easier for the individual.

(46) (B) Distracting themselves with objects and breathing to calm down.

Individuals use coping strategies to help remove negative feelings and brace themselves when problem behavior is shown. These may be consciously or unconsciously done to achieve the result and can vary depending on the situation.

Coping strategies include listening to music or taking long breaths to calm the mind.

(47) (D) Assisting with a replacement behavior.

Functional communication involves an individual socializing and communicating their needs. It helps effectively execute replacement behavior and allows a smoother transition.

(48) (B) Withdrawing reinforcement to discourage negative behavior.

To limit undesirable or negative behavior, it is necessary to engage in extinction. This process stops all reinforcement and eventually, the behavior comes to a halt.

(49) (C) By carefully assessing the situation or moving away.

The process of withholding reinforcement is carried out in various ways. Some technicians choose to practice methods such as trying to dissolve the situation by observing closely or distancing themselves when undesirable behavior occurs.

(50) (A) A child screaming when he wants ice cream.

People who want access to things act in various ways, showing different behaviors. If the action gives the child what he wants, he will just repeat it, as he believes it is the key to getting things in the future.

Access to tangibles is a function that refers to getting certain items or engaging in some enjoyable activity. Access-maintained behavior does not include direct actions. It can also be just looking at something the child wants or looking at the caregiver in a specific manner.

(51) (D) It helps the RBT identify why particular behavior occurs.

Functional behavior assessments allow the RBT to identify areas of concern and diagnose behavioral issues. They are also essential when choosing replacement behaviors.

(52) (C) Use different methods and observe their feelings.

Autism affects people differently, and some clients may find it difficult to transition from one task to another properly. So, it is important to use various methods to aid clients through this process and reduce any stress or anxiety. However, this is not true for all clients with ASD; sometimes stability in the environment may be needed.

(53) (A) Because it is covert or appears in the form of feelings.

Any action or communication is defined as behavior. However, there are instances when a behavior is not visible. These behaviors are referred to as covert behaviors and cannot be observed directly, such as being sad but not crying.

(54) (B) A teenager running away from home.

When an individual tries to remove themselves from a situation they do not want to be in, the action is referred to as escapism.

A teenager running away may indicate feelings of escapism. Perhaps the teenager wants to distance himself or herself from something undesirable at home.

Section 5: Documentation and Reporting

(55) (D) Admit to the supervisor immediately that you do not know how to use the strategy and ask to be shown how you do it.

RBTs must quickly inform their supervisor if they do not know how to implement a technique or strategy. There is no shame in that because you are there to learn. Your primary duty as an RBT is to complete all tasks appropriately.

(56) (A) A BCBA who is also an RBT supervisor.

Organizations with several RBTs and RBT supervisors name one individual to act as a coordinator for RBT requirements.

The organization's compliance with all supervision requirements is the responsibility of the RBT requirements coordinator. The RBT supervisor might also be the RBT requirements coordinator.

(57) (D) All of the above.

RBTs must gather information, note behavioral occurrences and provide session notes. Taking notes objectively and professionally is crucial while working with clients.

Factual observations and data gathered during and revealed by the client's evaluation are included in the objective notes.

The client's environment and how it might have affected their behavior throughout the session can also be mentioned in the session notes. However, it is important to have an objective stance when considering these factors.

(58) (B) Protect the passwords used to access the computer and spreadsheet program.

It is sometimes necessary to utilize electronic data logging programs because they are more efficient and accurate. However, to ensure privacy and data security, make sure your electronic footprint is protected with passwords.

Any information about the client should be kept private. Family members should not be given access to this information.

(59) (B) The client's dignity.

Everyone has a right to be treated with respect and dignity. So, as an RBT, consider your attitude, demeanor, compassion and communication to maintain client dignity and treat individuals with respect.

(60) (D) Marketing the agency.

Marketing the agency is not a part of the ethical code; spreading awareness of the ethics code, however, is. The ethics requirements are laid out in the RBT® Ethics Code (2.0). It offers specific advice for each of the three components: responsible behavior, duty to clients and competence and service delivery.

(61) (C) You should be familiar with the functions and definitions of the response you will be gauging during your session. Additionally, ensure you have everything you will need to collect data, including pens, paper and pencils.

Session notes and preparation are crucial before every session. You should be equipped with everything you need to conduct your lesson properly.

(62) (D) All of the above.

Once RBTs learn a client's rights are being violated, they should discuss their findings with the supervisor or another competent person. They must also distinguish between issues that require immediate attention and those that do not.

(63) (A) Justifying your actions because the supervisor could be mistaken in his or her feedback.

RBTs who receive effective supervisor feedback are supposed to reflect on their learning and learning practices. That process does not include justifying your actions because you think you are right.

Feedback can also be related to appropriate and inappropriate behavior and complying with the laws, regulations or standards of proper behavior or practice.

(64) (B) 5.

At least 5 percent of an RBT's total direct hours worked each month must be supervised.

Section 6: Professional Conduct and Scope of Practice

(65) (A) The RBT should interact with this client the same way she does with others.

RBTs' personal beliefs should not influence how they treat their clients or the clients' families.

For instance, if an RBT has issues with someone concerning smoking and observes one of her client's family members is smoking, she should treat the client the same way she treats others. She should never discriminate against a client.

(66) (B) It is not ethical under any circumstances.

It is not ethical for RBTs to have random conversations with their coworkers about their clients. So, they must not engage in small talk that reveals data about a client.

Client data could be as simple as a client's name or address. Discussions are discouraged even if a coworker knows the client.

(67) (A) Instantly inform the BCBA.

If RBTs realize that untrue information has been provided, they must instantly inform the BCBA.

(68) (D) 30 days.

RBTs should be aware of where the self-report needs to be sent. They should also know which events need self-report. The self-reporting process should be completed within 30 days of learning that certain events need to be self-reported.

The types of events that require self-reporting impact the RBT's ability to provide services. This can include an investigation by employees and institutions or legal charges against an RBT.

(69) (A) Eight.

People who supervise RBTs need to complete an eight-hour training based on the Supervisor Curriculum Training Outline.

(70) (D) He should notify his supervisor and concerned authorities.

If an RBT experiences issues concerning a client's behavior, he needs to notify his supervisors and concerned authorities. He is not allowed to make aggressive remarks toward clients, lose his temper or say anything that might hurt clients.

So, in this case, Derek should keep his expression neutral and inform his supervisor of the situation.

(71) (C) RBTs can share their clients' information only after gaining consent.

After getting consent, RBTs can share their clients' information with supervisors.

When securing information regarding sessions, RBTs need to ensure all information is safe. The data must be password protected and locked if it exists in a physical form.

(72) (A) RBTs should not discuss client-specific information with family.

RBTs should not discuss their clients' information with family members. They must protect their clients' data at all times.

(73) (A) It is unprofessional because it will create a bond between John and his clients.

RBTs should know that sharing links to their social media accounts is not a professional approach to treatment. Social media platforms reveal a person's personal life, and sharing them with clients will create an emotional bond, resulting in unprofessional behavior.

(74) (D) It shows a lack of professionalism.

To remain professional, RBTs must avoid giving advice to the client's family, friends or relatives.

(75) (D) They need to acquire consent before proceeding with the session.

RBTs must remember that before any conversation takes place, they need to acquire consent. Without consent, the conversation cannot be started.

In addition, RBTs need to remember to be precise and professional. They must not discourage the stakeholders' work or condemn them for anything during communication.

(76) (B) Use a token economy system.

This system is effective for children with ASD as it provides a clear and tangible reward for social initiatives. A token system allows for flexibility in rewards, which increases the chances that a desired behavior will be repeated.

(77) (A) Establish a baseline of her current money management skills.

Before an RBT teaches new skills to clients, it is essential to understand the learner's current abilities. A baseline allows for tailored instruction that meets the learner at her level of understanding. This step is critical to measure progress and adapt strategies to the learner's own needs.

(78) (A) Task analysis.

An RBT can break down complex tasks into smaller steps to simplify learning. This is especially true for individuals with developmental disabilities. Task analysis allows for focused instruction on each step, which makes it easier for the learner to acquire and master the skill.

(79) (B) Create a visual schedule and checklist for daily and weekly tasks.

Visual supports suit the learner's strengths and provide organized cues that guide task completion. This strategy improves independence in organizational tasks and leverages visual cues to compensate for attentional challenges common in ADHD.

(80) (A) Integrate social stories and interactive play as part of the consequences for correct responses.

An RBT can incorporate interests into education to maximize engagement and reinforce learning. Social stories and interactive play not only make the learning process enjoyable but also ensure that reinforcement is directly linked to the acquisition of targeted vocabulary.

(81) (A) Use communication cards to request a break.

Communication cards help the child express their needs in a socially acceptable manner. They are a direct and measurable approach that provides a clear alternative to inappropriate behavior.

(82) (C) Reward the child when they raise their hand to speak.

This method directly addresses the function of the behavior as it provides reinforcement for an appropriate behavior. It encourages the child to seek attention in a socially acceptable way.

(83) (C) Provide a stress ball as an alternative.

A stress ball can be a great way to address the sensory need that hand-flapping serves in a less disruptive manner. This method promotes the replacement of an undesirable behavior with a more appropriate one that fulfills the same need.

(84) (C) Increase the frequency of physical activity breaks.

This strategy addresses the possible sensory or escape-driven function that makes the client leave their seat and provides a structured alternative.

(85) (A) Ask peers for a turn with the toy.

A child must learn to request a turn instead of engaging in unwanted behavior. They should replace inappropriate behavior with positive behavior, which promotes skill acquisition in social interaction and reduces grab-related conflicts.

Test 3

Section 1: Measurement

(1) When measuring the duration of behavior, which of the following tools is used to gather data?

(A) Token.

(B) Scatterplot.

(C) Clicker.

(D) Stopwatch or timer.

(2) Which behavior demonstrates that Olivia is frustrated?

(A) Olivia is screaming "No!" during the session.

(B) Olivia is annoyed with her task.

(C) Olivia is sad.

(D) Olivia has a stomachache.

(3) Which of the following are basic sources of information depicted through a graph?

(A) Trend, variability, level.

(B) Contingency, level, reinforcement.

(C) X-axis, y-axis, hypotenuse.

(D) Level, slope, contingency.

(4) Deanna is a five-year-old who likes sucking her thumb. Her parents have asked the BCBA to help minimize her habit. The BCBA has asked you to gather baseline data.

Which measuring aspect would the BCBA find most helpful when creating an intervention plan?

(A) Rate.

(B) Frequency.

(C) Duration.

(D) Latency.

(5) Latency can be defined as _______.

(A) The number of responses.

(B) The frequency of occurrences.

(C) A measure of the time of each occurrence in every interval.

(D) The interval between the stimulus's presentation and the response it prompts.

(6) An RBT is supposed to record the data collected after running the permanent product procedure. The BCBA asked the RBT to input the data into a data table.

Why is this necessary?

(A) To understand the relationship between time and occurrences.

(B) To regress the data.

(C) To visually analyze data.

(D) To plot graphs and improve the efficiency of data collection.

(7) Which of the following are types of continuous measurement?

(A) Latency, momentary, duration.

(B) Duration, momentary, frequency.

(C) Frequency, whole-interval, duration.

(D) Frequency, rate, inter-response.

(8) Your supervisor instructs you to use partial interval recording in your sessions. Also, you have been tasked with recording a client's nail-biting in five-minute intervals while observing her for one hour.

How do you interpret this information?

(A) If the nail biting happens at any point throughout each five-minute interval, you will mark it as occurred.

(B) If the nail biting happened for the entire five-minute period, you will mark it as occurred.

(C) If the nail biting happened at the end of each five-minute period, you will mark it as occurred.

(D) If the nail biting did not happen during each five-minute period, you will mark it as occurred.

(9) Alice is a 15-year-old girl with an eating disorder. You are analyzing her relationship with food and eating habits. Using a type of continuous measurement method, you record that Alice takes five minutes between bites of food.

What did you record?

(A) Inter-response time.

(B) Latency.

(C) Permanent product.

(D) Duration.

(10) Data-gathering is an essential component of behavior analysis because __________.

(A) It enables data-driven decisions.

(B) It allows tracking of development and the identification of skill gaps.

(C) It aids in determining skill mastery.

(D) All of the above.

(11) Oksana does not concentrate in class. Her teacher wants to improve her concentration and asks for help from an RBT. The RBT had a session with Oksana in a playground and recorded all necessary data. However, the BCBA stated that the data was unreliable.

In your opinion, which crucial step of task analysis did the RBT not implement?

(A) Holding the session in the playground.

(B) Determining the type of behavior.

(C) Choosing the best data collection method.

(D) Eliminating distractions.

(12) Which item is not needed if you intend to make a frequency recording of Peter whistling during a group meeting?

(A) A timer.

(B) A whole-interval datasheet.

(C) A pen.

(D) A calculator.

Section 2: Assessment

(13) What is not an advantage of the indirect functional behavior assessment?

(A) It acts as a source of information in guiding more objective assessments.

(B) It helps generate hypotheses about variables that cannot be observed during direct observation.

(C) It is considered convenient by many people.

(D) It generates unbiased data for subsequent assessments.

(14) An RBT is conducting a preference assessment with Sara. The RBT presents eight items in one array simultaneously. Sara chooses gum out of the variety. However, instead of letting Sara consume it, the RBT puts the chosen item back in the presentation.

The RBT collects data on the number of trials in which the item is selected relative to the number of trials in which it was presented. What kind of preference assessment is this?

(A) Multiple stimulus with replacement.

(B) Paired stimulus.

(C) Single stimulus.

(D) Multiple stimulus without replacement.

(15) Jeremiah's parents asked him to get off his computer, but he refused to leave his desk and screamed "NO!" five times. A few minutes later, Jeremiah's mom asked him to step away from his computer again and gave him a 10-second warning.

According to the ABC data collection model, what is the antecedent in the example?

(A) Jeremiah's mom asked Jeremiah to leave his computer again and gave him a 10-second warning.

(B) Jeremiah refused to leave his place and screamed "NO!" five times.

(C) Jeremiah's parents asked him to get off his computer.

(D) None of the above.

(16) ______ is a systematic assessment of the antecedents and consequences that tell us why the target behavior occurs.

(A) Indirect assessment.

(B) Functional analysis.

(C) Functional behavior assessment.

(D) Direct assessment.

(17) One item is presented at a time in a behavioral assessment. The RBT notes down if the client approaches an item. In this preference assessment, hierarchy is based on how often the item was available versus how often it was approached.

This is an example of __________.

(A) Free-operant observation preference assessment.

(B) Single-stimulus preference assessment.

(C) Forced-choice preference assessment.

(D) Multiple-stimulus preference without replacement.

(18) The purpose of describing behavioral function is to clarify ________.

(A) How the behavior happens.

(B) For how long the behavior occurs.

(C) When the behavior occurs.

(D) Why the behavior occurs.

Section 3: Skill Acquisition

(19) Which of the following best describes a response difference in the presence of different stimuli?

(A) Stimulus control.

(B) General control.

(C) Behavioral control.

(D) Physical control.

(20) A student is very talkative with friends but remains silent in class. Which of the following is responsible for exerting stimulus control over the student?

(A) Social environment.

(B) Student.

(C) Friends.

(D) None of the above.

(21) Some techniques involve using discontinued prompts after target behavior has begun being displayed in the presence of a discriminative stimulus.

These techniques are called ________.

(A) Current stimulus.

(B) Hand signal.

(C) Transfer of stimulus.

(D) Stimulus-control transfer procedures.

(22) In cases where the client does not independently make the proper response to instructions, which of the following can be used?

(A) Prompting.

(B) Inter-trial period.

(C) Intrusiveness.

(D) Behavioral training.

(23) What are different types of gestural prompts?

(A) Full physical prompts, partial physical prompts, behavioral prompts and positional prompts.

(B) Delivering the instruction, waiting for a correct response, immediately recording data and regaining the learner's attention while presenting the next instruction.

(C) Full physical prompts, partial physical prompts, verbal prompts and positional prompts.

(D) Full physical prompts, verbal prompts, intrusive prompts and positional prompts.

(24) Which of the following best describes the most intrusive prompt and hand-over-hand assistance?

(A) Full physical prompts.

(B) Partial physical prompts.

(C) Verbal prompts.

(D) Positional prompts.

(25) Which of the following is a less intrusive method in which the instructor guides subjects through the part of the assigned activity?

(A) A full physical prompt.

(B) A partial physical prompt.

(C) A verbal prompt.

(D) A positional prompt.

(26) Which of the following prompts allows the learner to give the correct response?

(A) Full physical prompts.

(B) Partial physical prompts.

(C) Verbal prompts.

(D) Positional prompts.

(27) The removal of prompts combined with instruction allows the learner to perform independently. This is called ______.

(A) Prompt fading.

(B) Verbal prompt.

(C) Positional prompt.

(D) General prompt.

(28) What are the three main elements of prompt fading?

(A) Physical, positional delay, proximity.

(B) Physical, general, proximity.

(C) Physical, time delay, proximity.

(D) Physical, time delay, verbal.

(29) A trainer uses prompt fading that includes a decreasing level of intrusiveness. It is carried out by following an immediate hierarchy, using most to least prompting.

The trainer is using which of the following elements of prompt fading?

(A) Proximity.

(B) Time delay.

(C) Verbal.

(D) Physical.

(30) Which elements of prompt fading include introducing a systematic change in the learner's spatial positions?

(A) Physical.

(B) Time delay.

(C) Proximity.

(D) General.

(31) In generalization, an individual will apply something learned in a specific situation to a similar situation determined by progress toward the therapy goal. What is this called?

(A) Carryover.

(B) Proximity.

(C) Generalization.

(D) Time delay.

(32) What are several types of generalization methods?

(A) Teaching multiple examples, teaching across numerous people, training with various instructions, choosing functional behavior.

(B) Teaching multiple examples, behavioral teaching, teaching with various instructions, choosing functional behavior.

(C) Teaching multiple examples, teaching across numerous people, training with various instructions, physical teaching.

(D) Teaching multiple examples, teaching across numerous people, teaching with various instructions, inter-period teaching.

(33) A client has several different teachers. Which generalization method should the teachers choose?

(A) Teaching multiple examples.

(B) Teaching across multiple people.

(C) Teaching with multiple instructions.

(D) Choosing functional behavior.

(34) A client wants to get reinforcement from the environment independently. What generalization method should be used?

(A) Teaching multiple examples.

(B) Teaching across multiple people.

(C) Teaching with multiple instructions.

(D) Choosing functional behavior.

(35) Which of the following best describes continued skill performance after teaching has stopped?

(A) Functional behavior.

(B) Teaching across multiple people.

(C) Maintenance.

(D) Generalization.

(36) A process involves reinforcing the client whenever approximations of the desired behavior are shown. This is called _____.

(A) Shaping.

(B) Initial process.

(C) Functional behavior.

(D) Maintenance.

(37) In the initial process, why does the RBT need to know what behavior is required to be achieved?

(A) To teach the client the first step.

(B) To choose the target behavior.

(C) To determine the present performance level.

(D) To make it easier for the client to understand how things proceed.

(38) The shaping process involves an analysis in which the behavior is broken down into smaller steps that are easier to administer.

What is this analysis called?

(A) Task analysis.

(B) General analysis.

(C) Behavioral analysis.

(D) Random analysis.

(39) Which of the following involves the delivery of a tangible conditioned reinforcer using a contingency-based method to help decrease maladaptive behaviors?

(A) A random economy.

(B) A token economy.

(C) Frequency.

(D) A reinforcement strategy.

(40) Which of the following contains reinforcers for the token economy?

(A) Generalized reinforcers; general reinforcers.

(B) Generalized reinforcers; physical reinforcers.

(C) Generalized reinforcers; backup reinforcers.

(D) Backup reinforcers; physical reinforcers.

(41) What are rewards or tokens given by RBTs every time a client exhibits target behavior?

(A) Random economy.

(B) Generalized reinforcers.

(C) Backup reinforcers.

(D) Reinforcement strategy.

(42) A client knows that collecting rewards will give her access to another kind of reward. So, she repeats a certain behavior.

What is the most likely outcome of this scenario?

(A) The client learns to exhibit behavior independently without being reinforced.

(B) The client is reinforced.

(C) The client does not learn to exhibit the behavior independently.

(D) The client exhibits the behavior independently only when she is reinforced.

Section 4: Behavior Reduction

(43) When is the differential reinforcement of low rates procedure used?

(A) During an aggressive episode.

(B) For repeated behaviors.

(C) When behavior is appropriate.

(D) None of the above.

(44) What can be done to make a child choose good behavior practices?

(A) Give punishment.

(B) Offer comfort and motivation.

(C) Give less attention.

(D) Both (A) and (C).

(45) How many types of differential reinforcement exist?

(A) Four.

(B) Three.

(C) Two.

(D) One.

(46) Giving a child candy after he gets good grades on a test is an example of ________.

(A) Negative punishment.

(B) Positive reinforcement.

(C) Negative reinforcement.

(D) Positive punishment.

(47) Which of the following is an example of differential reinforcement of alternative behavior?

(A) A child is told to sit and wait but constantly runs around; as a result, he is not reinforced.

(B) A child screams and gets his point across.

(C) A child is being appreciated when he does the right thing even if it means going against the social acceptance of peers.

(D) None of the above.

(48) A technician stays silent when faced with undesirable behavior. What does this indicate about the technician?

(A) He is satisfied with the progress.

(B) He is avoiding reinforcement/ignoring the action.

(C) He is rewarding the action.

(D) He accepts the behavior.

(49) Adam is an average student. He receives an A on his math test, after which his teacher praises him in class. As a result, his level of studying decreases and his grades plummet.

Which of the following would explain this situation?

(A) Positive reinforcement.

(B) Negative punishment.

(C) Positive punishment.

(D) Reward.

(50) What happens when a person is rewarded for a certain action?

(A) He becomes aggressive.

(B) He will repeat that behavior.

(C) He will not fear punishment.

(D) He will crave attention.

(51) Who can create a behavior plan and what is it dependent on?

(A) Professionals, parents and peers; the seriousness of the issue.

(B) Professionals; the client's mood.

(C) Friends and family; their relationship with the client.

(D) Both (A) and (B).

(52) A woman gives her dog food every day after he obeys the command to sit. The dog learns to sit; however, when the woman stops giving food, the dog stops obeying the command or responding specifically to it.

This is an example of __________.

(A) Negative reinforcement.

(B) Preventive strategy.

(C) Identifying information.

(D) Spontaneous recovery.

(53) A proper guideline is established to avoid repeat occurrences of a certain behavior. Which of the following parts of a behavior plan does this come under?

(A) Consequence strategy.

(B) Preventive strategy.

(C) Identifying information.

(D) Data collection.

(54) What is the main goal for applying consequential strategies?

(A) To determine what should happen when behavior is unacceptable.

(B) To prevent problematic behavior.

(C) To gather information.

(D) Both (A) and (B).

Section 5: Documentation and Reporting

(55) Which of the following approaches is ideal for maintaining the confidentiality of session records in writing?

(A) Keep all notes in a binder with the materials for the intervention.

(B) Lock all notes in a filing cabinet.

(C) Place notes on desks inside work areas, away from clients.

(D) Keep notes and other paperwork in the administrative office.

(56) Which of the following best describes how frequently RBTs should contact their supervisors?

(A) RBTs should exclusively schedule communications with their supervisors.

(B) RBTs should consult with their supervisors as necessary.

(C) RBTs should keep in daily contact with their supervisors.

(D) RBTs should contact their supervisors when asked to do so.

(57) If an RBT believes a client has been mishandled or abused, she should __________.

(A) Examine the client and his behavior before informing the supervisor of her suspicions.

(B) Confront anyone she believes is mistreating the client before reporting her suspicions.

(C) Promptly inform law enforcement of her suspicions, regardless of the organization's policy.

(D) Immediately inform her supervisor of her suspicions in accordance with the organization's rules.

(58) Your supervisor assigns you to work with a new client who exhibits behaviors you are unfamiliar with.

What should you do?

(A) Refuse because you lack relevant experience.

(B) Ask the supervisory BCBA for additional training.

(C) Accept the assignment because you have a legal obligation to do so.

(D) Politely appeal the assignment.

(59) A client's guardians ask to speak with you after your session. They question how long your client will require behavioral therapy.

You should inform them that:

(A) You will go home and research their question.

(B) The BCBA or supervisor will contact them to discuss their question.

(C) Based on your experience, you believe the client will require two years of intensive therapy.

(D) They should stop asking questions.

(60) Reporting entails ___________.

(A) Writing session notes.

(B) Communicating with the BCBA on a case.

(C) Entering ABC data not included in the behavior intervention plan.

(D) All of the above.

(61) Samuel finds his client committing self-harm. He attempts to contact his supervisor after resolving the issue to the best of his ability but is unsuccessful because his supervisor is not immediately available via email.

Which of the following emails would be most objective?

(A) "Our meeting didn't go well. I require help! Can you please respond immediately?"

(B) "Today the client became furious and engaged in some SIB. Please help."

(C) "He wasn't acting like himself today."

(D) "The client banged his head repeatedly on the table for 30 seconds while making a loud 'aaa' sound. To curb the behavior, I set a pillow on the table. This behavior was new, according to the client's mother."

(62) Which of the following answers best describes RBTs' function in delivering behavioral services?

(A) If they have sufficient experience, RBTs can supervise other RBTs and, if their employer approves, design and implement behavior modification programs.

(B) RBTs can create and carry out behavior modification plans. The supervisor is supposed to assess their work once every three months and notify the BCBA of any violations.

(C) An RBT is a type of license. So, to keep their credentials, RBTs must complete 20 continuing-education units every two years after becoming licensed.

(D) A certified behavior technician's behavior reduction plan is implemented mainly by the BCBA. To ensure expertise, he or she receives regular supervision from a qualified analyst.

(63) You are advised to use MOO language in your session notes. MOO stands for ______.

(A) Measurable, observable, objective.

(B) Maintained original, on-point.

(C) Maintenance, operant, objective.

(D) Momentary original, observable.

(64) The difference between a BCBA and RBT is that __________.

(A) A BCBA can practice independently.

(B) A BCBA can be the supervisor of an RBT.

(C) An RBT can practice independently.

(D) Both A and B.

Section 6: Professional Conduct and Scope of Practice

(65) Which of the following includes credentials approved by the BCBA?

(A) BCBA-E, BCBA, BCaBA, RBT.

(B) BCBA-D, BCBA, BCaBA, RBT.

(C) BCBA-A, BCBA, BCaBA, RBT.

(D) BCBA-E, BCBA, BCaBB, RBT.

(66) What is the RBT's responsibility when a supervisor gives feedback?

(A) The RBT should comply with the feedback.

(B) The RBT should ignore the feedback.

(C) The RBT is not responsible for following the feedback.

(D) None of the above.

(67) Misusing confidential information belonging to a supervisor has detrimental effects. Why is that?

(A) Because it contains data from the client's family.

(B) Because it includes communication logs.

(C) Because it includes certification titles and examination content.

(D) Because it features the BCBA's information.

(68) Who are the client's stakeholders?

(A) Family, caregivers and other professionals.

(B) The supervisor.

(C) The supervisor's family.

(D) The RBT.

(69) When giving feedback, what should supervisors keep in mind about improving RBT skills?

(A) RBTs need to improve their skills immediately.

(B) RBTs are unable to improve their skills.

(C) Feedback will not help RBTs improve their skills.

(D) Enhancing skills takes time and cannot be done immediately.

(70) Why should an RBT involve the client's family in the process?

(A) It is mandated by law.

(B) The client's family can analyze what can be done to help the client.

(C) RBTs should not involve the client's family.

(D) Involving the client's family will not help the client.

(71) Why is personally developing a system for documenting supervising experience allowed for supervisors?

(A) It allows for an individualized perspective of supervisory notes.

(B) It is a requirement of the client.

(C) It is a requirement of the client's family.

(D) It is beneficial for the RBT.

(72) What is the minimum percentage of hours the RBT must obtain supervision for offering their services?

(A) 8 percent.

(B) 7 percent.

(C) 6 percent.

(D) 5 percent.

(73) Why must the RBT supervisor be able to describe outcomes and strategies regarding ineffective supervision?

(A) It is a requirement of the client's family.

(B) It is a requirement of the RBT's family.

(C) It is a legal requirement of the RBT.

(D) It is necessary to evaluate insufficient client progress, poor performance and unethical behavior.

(74) A supervisor evaluates an RBT's strengths and weaknesses.

What is the purpose of this evaluation?

(A) It can improve the RBT's performance.

(B) It is a requirement of the client.

(C) It is mandated by law.

(D) It motivates the RBT.

(75) How can empathy help RBTs develop a better relationship with their clients?

(A) It can allow them to understand what a client's family is feeling.

(B) It helps them become more compassionate toward every person who struggles with problematic behaviors.

(C) It allows them to understand the clients' problems and help deal with them.

(D) None of the above.

(76) An RBT works under the supervision of a BCBA and is required to document each session's outcomes and strategies. Which of these is the most important aspect for the RBT to include in their session notes?

(A) The client's mood and general observations.

(B) Specific behaviors observed, interventions used, and the client's response.

(C) Personal opinions on the client's progress.

(D) Plans for the next session.

(77) A BCBA reviews an RBT's performance during a monthly supervision session. What aspect of the RBT's work should the BCBA focus on for quality improvement?

(A) The RBT's ability to engage in small talk with clients.

(B) Adherence to ethical guidelines and accurate data collection.

(C) The RBT's feelings about the success of interventions.

(D) The RBT's preferences for certain types of interventions over others.

(78) An RBT encounters a new behavior from a client that was not previously observed. What action should they take first?

(A) Discuss the behavior with colleagues for their opinion.

(B) Implement a new intervention plan right away.

(C) Document the behavior and report it to the BCBA supervisor.

(D) Ignore the behavior until it becomes frequent.

(79) A BCBA assigns a new RBT to observe sessions and provide feedback. What is a key element that the RBT should focus on during observations?

(A) The client's family dynamics and home environment.

(B) The BCBA's style of communication with the client.

(C) Accurate documentation of the client's behavior and the interventions used.

(D) The comfort level of the client's family with the BCBA.

(80) An RBT needs to communicate a significant change in a client's behavior to her supervisor. What is the most effective way to ensure the communication is clear and actionable?

(A) Send a brief text message to the BCBA.

(B) Prepare a detailed report that includes the behavior, context, and any interventions attempted.

(C) Wait for the next scheduled supervision meeting to meet face-to-face.

(D) Discuss it informally with the BCBA during a break.

(81) An RBT prepares for their first supervision session with a new BCBA supervisor. The RBT wants to demonstrate professionalism and readiness. What is the next most appropriate action?

(A) Bring a list of personal achievements in ABA therapy to discuss.

(B) Prepare a summary of recent client sessions.

(C) Request from the supervisor to handle difficult cases.

(D) Avoid discussing any challenges to appear more competent.

(82) During a supervision session, the BCBA supervisor notices that the RBT consistently struggles to implement a specific intervention. What is the most appropriate next step for the supervisor?

(A) Reassign the RBT to less challenging clients.

(B) Schedule extra unpaid hours for the RBT to practice the intervention.

(C) Demonstrate the intervention, observe the RBT's application, and provide feedback.

(D) Advise the RBT to review the intervention protocol on their own time.

(83) An RBT receives feedback from their supervisor that suggests areas for improvement. The RBT feels defensive and considers how to respond. What is the best approach?

(A) Dismiss the feedback respectfully.

(B) Accept the feedback and ask for clarification.

(C) Request a transfer to a different supervisor who may have a more favorable opinion.

(D) Ignore the feedback and continue with their current practice.

(84) A BCBA supervisor plans the structure of supervision for an RBT. Which element is essential to include in their plan?

(A) Ensure that all supervision occurs in group settings to facilitate peer learning.

(B) Observe the RBT with a client at least once a month to provide direct feedback.

(C) Limit feedback to written reports to streamline the supervision process.

(D) Focus on the RBT's strengths to boost confidence and morale.

(85) An RBT wants to build a positive supervisory relationship with their BCBA. What action by the RBT would most effectively contribute to this goal?

(A) Focus on personal interests to make the supervision more enjoyable.

(B) Communicate progress and challenges.

(C) Avoid discussing any mistakes made during sessions.

(D) Insist on less supervision time.

Test 3: Answers and Explanations

Section 1: Measurement

(1) (D) Stopwatch or timer.

Duration is the time or period during which a behavior occurs. The most essential tool you require is a stopwatch or timer to record data.

(2) (A) Olivia is screaming “No!” during the session.

Behavior is defined as an act that is both observable and measurable. Emotions or feelings are not considered behaviors in behavioral science.

The RBT can measure the frequency of Olivia saying no and observe it. Similarly, anger and annoyance are emotions that need to be reflected in a measurable behavior. RBT cannot observe if Olivia has a stomachache.

(3) (A) Trend, variability, level.

Behavior analysts mainly refer to a graph’s trend, level and variability. On a graph, trend refers to the general flow of the data. Usual trend labels include increasing, decreasing and zero.

The position of the data on the vertical axis is defined as the level of data points. Behavior levels can generally be classified as low, moderate or high. The range of deviation of the data points around the line serves as a measure of variability. It demands an evaluation of the data after several sessions.

In ABA, variability is typically interpreted by drawing a best-fit line through the data points. The variability is low if a large number of data points are near the line. However, variability is high if numerous data points significantly depart from that line.

(4) (C) Duration.

Data from the baseline serves as a place to start. The BCBA can create an intervention to lessen thumb-sucking once he or she knows how much time Deanna spends doing it. The BCBA can be certain that the intervention is effective only if the facts support it.

Although other responses might be useful, they would not be as beneficial to the effort to lessen thumb-sucking as a baseline.

(5) (D) The interval between the stimulus's presentation and the response it prompts.

Latency is a type of continuous measurement procedure. Systems for collecting continuous measurement data keep track of each instance of a target behavior. Examples of common continuous measuring techniques include frequency, inter-response time and duration.

The period between the presentation of a stimulus and the onset of behavior is known as latency. The frequency, rate and percentage of time measure how frequently the behavior occurs based on the number of responses counted, the number of responses per unit of time and the number of responses per second.

An example of latency is how long it takes for a student to start responding after being given a question.

(6) (D) To plot graphs and improve the efficiency of data collection.

To ensure that data is organized and ready for plotting, each graph must contain a data table. The use of graphed data is essential because it supports the process of visual-based instructional decision-making and aids in conveying information about the observation. Furthermore, the graph demonstrates a relationship or link between the dependent and independent variables.

(7) (D) Frequency, rate, inter-response.

In ABA, continuous measurement tracks every instance of behavior throughout a lesson, session or day. An RBT should understand the following continuous measurement terms: frequency, rate, duration, IRT (inter-response time) and latency.

The length of time between an antecedent (such as a teacher's instruction) and the moment the student starts to carry out a specific behavior is measured by latency recording.

In contrast, the inter-response time is the period between two instances of an activity that occur back to back, and the frequency of the behavior in a time is referred to as its rate.

(8) (A) If nail biting happens at any point throughout each five-minute interval, you will mark it as occurred.

In a partial interval recording, you record if a behavior occurs at any point within the given interval. If a behavior occurs during the interval, you record it by marking it with an X for occurrence and an O for no occurrence.

For an X to be recorded, a client may exhibit behavior more than once within the period or only once. For example, if the client in this case bites her nails once or more during the five-minute period, you will mark it as occurring.

In the case of whole interval recording, the RBT would have recorded it if the nail biting had happened for the entire five-minute period. Moreover, he would have recorded if the activity was happening at the end of each five-minute period if he was conducting momentary time sampling.

(9) (A) Inter-response time.

The interval between two responses is known as the inter-response time. It is important to note that these two responses occur in the same interval or session.

The IRT is five minutes if Alice waits five minutes between bites. Similarly, the IRT is 10 hours if she takes 10-hour-long breaks between meals.

(10) (D) All of the above.

Data collection is crucial from the RBT's point of view because it aids in documenting the client's successes and allows the RBT to spot new behaviors in the client. This may make it easier to determine whether the therapy being utilized has a favorable or unfavorable effect.

(11) (D) Eliminating distractions.

The technician must manage the environment and remove unnecessary variables for a reliable assessment and analysis. A noisy room or playground might be an example of an unnecessary variable.

In the question, the data provided by the RBT became unreliable because the RBT did not ensure the client was not being influenced by other variables, like playground noise.

(12) (B) A whole-interval datasheet.

Frequency recording is a type of continuous measurement. It happens when you count the number of times a behavior occurs throughout a session.

In comparison, a whole-data interval is a type of discontinuous measurement. It happens when a behavior occurs throughout a predetermined time interval. As a result, you will not need a whole datasheet for frequency data recording.

Section 2: Assessment

(13) (D) It generates unbiased data for subsequent assessments.

The indirect functional behavior assessment acts as a source of information in guiding later, more objective assessments; helps generate hypotheses about a variable that cannot be observed during direct observation; and is considered convenient by many people.

However, it may provide inaccurate data because people being interviewed may be biased. The rate scales can also produce results with a poor inter-rate agreement.

(14) (D) Multiple stimulus without replacement.

During multiple stimulus without replacement assessments, the RBT provides the client with an array of items (often toys or sweets) and asks him to choose one. The RBT takes the item out of the collection after the client uses or consumes it. The RBT notes the array's items and the client's choice of each one in the array's order.

However, in the multiple stimulus with replacement preference assessment, the RBT presents the client with various items (usually toys or edibles) and allows him to choose one. After the client uses or consumes the item, the RBT replaces it in the array and substitutes the unselected items with new ones.

Similarly, in paired-stimulus preference assessments, stimuli are presented in pairs until every other stimulus has been presented with one another. Then the hierarchy of preferences is generated.

Single-stimulus preference assessments are carried out by giving a client a single item and observing the behavior and amount of time spent engaging with each item.

(15) (C) Jeremiah's parents asked him to get off his computer.

A behavior implementation plan should be developed from the information gathered on an ABC data form, which is a tool for assessment.

According to ABC, things that happen, take place or are in place before conduct are called antecedents; behavior occurs in response to the antecedent; consequences are the action or reaction that results from a behavior.

So, the antecedent in this situation is Jeremiah's parents asking him to get off his computer.

(16) (C) Functional behavior assessment.

A functional behavior assessment aims to ascertain the function of the target behavior by conducting a systematic analysis of the antecedents and outcomes of the target behavior. There are two types of functional behavior assessments: indirect and direct assessments.

(17) (B) Single-stimulus preference assessment.

One item is presented at a time in a single-stimulus preference assessment. If the client chooses the item, the RBT records the action. The hierarchy is determined by how frequently an item was available compared to how often it was approached.

(18) (D) Why the behavior occurs.

A functional behavioral assessment determines the cause behind a client's problematic behavior. The method's objective is to identify the antecedent of troublesome behavior and find potential solutions for it.

To determine the purpose of the troublesome behavior, RBTs use direct assessment techniques—including descriptive assessment—to observe and gather data about antecedents, behavior and outcomes. This process is frequently referred to as collecting ABC data.

Section 3: Skill Acquisition

(19) (A) Stimulus control.

In everyday life, behaviors involve stimulus control in some way or another. Stimulus control is a difference in responding in the presence of various stimuli. It occurs when an individual behaves in one way in sight of one given stimulus and another in its absence.

A typical example is a driver putting his foot on the brake pedal to respond to a red light. The same driver puts his foot on the accelerator when the light turns green. Therefore, the driver's response is under stimulus control of the traffic light's color.

Stimulus control is central to comprehending normal and abnormal behavior. It helps to generate behavior guidelines for studying the effects of drugs and other physical implications.

(20) (A) Social environment.

The stimulus control is responsible for either encouraging or obstructing behavior. An example is a student who might be very talkative with friends but remains quiet in class.

In this case, the social environment with friends encourages the student to talk, while the environment in the school inhibits talking behavior. Therefore, the student's social environment exerts stimulus control over her behavior.

(21) (D) Stimulus-control transfer procedures.

Techniques that involve discontinuing prompts after target behavior has started in the presence of a discriminative stimulus are known as stimulus control transfer procedures. Such procedures link discriminative stimulus with action and add another stimulus that leads to the same activity.

The transfer of stimulus control involves changing cues. For example, if the initial cue is a spoken command, it can be later changed to a hand signal. The cue can be paired with a task or instruction.

An RBT can use the cue with the discriminative stimulus or the instructional materials. When the stimulus is absent, the behavior is put on extinction or ignored.

(22) (A) Prompting.

Clients sometimes do not produce correct responses or independently make proper responses to instructions or commons. This can happen in learning new skills and such instances require prompting.

Cues, along with instruction, can increase the likelihood of students producing accurate responses, known as prompting. When a client has access to reinforcement for responding accurately, the chance of behavior occurring more often increases.

So, prompting is beneficial for teaching new skills. This includes the most intrusive level of prompt necessary for students' success.

(23) (C) Full physical prompts, partial physical prompts, verbal prompts and positional prompts.

A gestural prompt includes gestures or any action the client can observe. It may consist of nodding, reaching, pointing or any action that gives information about an accurate response.

There are four types of gestural prompts, including full physical prompts, partial physical prompts, verbal prompts and positional prompts.

(24) (A) Full physical prompts.

Full physical prompts include physically helping the client complete the task. These are thought to be the most intrusive prompt and are also known as hand-over-hand assistance.

(25) (B) A partial physical prompt.

The RBT assists the client through part of the given activity with partial physical prompts. This is a less intrusive method compared to a physical prompt.

For instance, an RBT teaches a client how to use a spoon to eat. She uses partial physical prompts and moves the client's hand toward a spoon.

(26) (D) Positional prompts.

When using positional prompts, the trainer places the accurate response closest to learners to give them information. An example is a teacher showing the student three objects: a toy, a shoe and an orange.

The teacher says, "Point your finger toward the one you wear." She then places the shoe near the child. In this scenario, the teacher has put the correct response—the shoe—near the child. It serves as a positional prompt.

(27) (A) Prompt fading.

The reduction of prompts paired with instruction is known as prompt fading. It enables learners to perform independently. This procedure prevents learners from being dependent on prompts and includes removing prompts quickly.

(28) (C) Physical, time delay, proximity.

Prompt fading includes physical, time delay and proximity prompts. A complete physical prompt is faded to a partial physical prompt. It includes reducing intrusiveness, which is done by following an immediate hierarchy using most to least prompting.

Time delay includes increasing the use of prompts by slowly increasing the time between delivery time and instruction, and proximity includes introducing a structured change in the learner's spatial positions.

(29) (D) Physical.

A complete physical prompt involves reducing intrusiveness, which is done by following a prompt hierarchy using most to least prompting. The prompt includes physically helping the learner achieve the target behavior.

For instance, a parent could tap the toddler's hand, which is already on the toy car, to signal him to climb into the car. The RBT uses these prompts when the learner does not accurately respond to less restrictive prompts.

(30) (C) Proximity.

The proximity prompt includes introducing a systematic change in the learner's spatial positions.

(31) (A) Carryover.

In generalization, the learner applies something in a particular situation to similar situations marked by progress toward the therapy goal. This is known as carryover. It applies to incidents in which the trainer sees the client's progress outside the therapy environment, such as school, parks, etc.

Carryover can include several people, such as parents or teachers. The procedure is not automatic and needs constant work to ensure fruitful behavior change.

(32) (A) Teaching multiple examples, teaching across numerous people, training with various instructions, choosing functional behavior.

Generalization methods include teaching multiple examples, teaching across numerous people, training with multiple instructions and choosing a functional behavior.

The teaching multiple examples strategy is one of the most reliable ways of generalization and is applied across different settings. When various people teach clients, the instruction will ensure clients learn to act with several people.

In contrast, the teaching with multiple instructions strategy is used for clients with autism, as learning and understanding different instructions can be complicated. The RBT begins by teaching one skill, followed by another, which is constantly reinforced.

(33) (B) Teaching across multiple people.

The teaching across multiple people method is most effective if a client has a different teacher. When several people teach the client, their training will allow them to interact with different people.

(34) (D) Choosing functional behavior.

Choosing functional behavior allows learners to be taught behavior that is beneficial in everyday life. It allows them to get reinforcement from the environment as well.

(35) (C) Maintenance.

Continued performance of a specific skill after teaching has halted is known as maintenance. Maintenance happens if a client exhibits a particular behavior after the teaching process for it has stopped.

Simply put, maintenance can be identified as the client's ability to demonstrate obtained skills over time.

(36) (A) Shaping.

In ABA, shaping is the reinforcement of successive approximations of desired behavior. The process includes reinforcing the client whenever an approximation of desired behavior is exhibited.

The client will not be reinforced if the RBT does not perform the approximations of the desired behavior. Experts also define shaping as a process in which the trainer teaches a behavioral skill to the client. So, the RBT gives reinforcement whenever the learner performs the desired behavior. This reinforcement helps teach new skills, as it is a component of behavior analysis.

However, defining the behavioral objective is essential for shaping to be effective and successful. RBTs must know when to reinforce clients and when to withhold reinforcement. Before using shaping, they must also consider their knowledge of the clients and their behaviors.

(37) (D) To make it easier for the client to understand how things proceed.

Before the actual procedure begins, the RBT performs a few steps to ensure the best possible outcome. However, before doing that, the RBT needs to know what behavior is required to be achieved.

The steps taken by the RBT make it easier for the client to comprehend how things develop.

(38) (A) Task analysis.

The shaping process begins with a task analysis. It involves desired behavior broken down into simpler steps that are easier to administer. The analysis aims to bring the client closer to the desired behavior.

The desired behavior is an example of working independently for five minutes; task analysis will break target behavior into smaller steps. Some steps could be working for four minutes with two prompts, working for eight minutes with a maximum of two prompts and so on.

(39) (B) A token economy.

A token economy is a contingency-based method created to reduce maladaptive behaviors. It increases desired behaviors through a tangible conditioned reinforcer.

A generalized conditional reinforcer is one specific reinforcer associated with at least two or more backup reinforcers. Backup reinforcers are real objects or activities that act as a reinforcer for the learner. Moreover, a generalized conditional reinforcer does not have to be an actual item but can include more natural forms of reinforcement.

Token economies use a tangible representation of generalized conditioned reinforcers. Some examples of tokens are poker chips, marbles, color chars, Legos, etc.

(40) (C) Generalized reinforcers; backup reinforcers.

Generalized reinforcers are rewards the RBT gives every time the learner exhibits the target behavior. The client can collect the tokens and exchange them with backup reinforcers.

Backup reinforcers are rewards clients get by exchanging collected tokens, such as treats, snacks or candies.

(41) (B) Generalized reinforcers.

Generalized reinforcers are tokens given by RBT every time the learner accurately exhibits target behavior.

(42) (A) The client learns to exhibit behavior independently without being reinforced.

When clients know collecting rewards will give them the opportunity for another kind of reward, the clients may repeat the behavior. They may also learn to exhibit the behavior independently without being reinforced.

Reinforcement is unnecessary, as the clients will continue to repeat the behavior until they get the reward.

Section 4: Behavior Reduction

(43) (B) For repeated behaviors.

Differential reinforcement of low rates is used for repeated behaviors that appear too often. This may become unhealthy, so technicians consider using DRL, which focuses on such actions.

(44) (B) Offer comfort and motivation.

Appropriate behavior should be praised and given more attention. If a proper list of tasks is given and the place of the learning is comfortable, then the child will choose appropriate and desirable behavior more. The process should motivate the child.

(45) (A) Four.

There are four types of differential reinforcement.

(46) (B) Positive reinforcement.

Positive reinforcement refers to introducing a desirable stimulus after a behavior. It reinforces the behavior and makes it more likely that the behavior will reoccur in the future.

(47) (A) A child is told to sit and wait but constantly runs around; as a result, he is not reinforced.

In the differential reinforcement of alternative behavior, certain actions are reinforced to avoid the problem behavior.

In this procedure, the problem behavior and the alternative can sometimes occur simultaneously. However, the acknowledgment should be given only to the latter, since it is socially conforming.

So, when the child is not obeying the action, he should not be given what he wants until he sits down and waits.

(48) (B) He is avoiding reinforcement/ignoring the action.

When inappropriate behavior is shown, reinforcement is stopped. The technician can ignore these unacceptable actions. This may be done in different ways, including distancing himself from the place, staying silent, etc.

(49) (C) Positive punishment.

The main purpose of positive punishment is to reduce the future occurrence of inappropriate behavior by applying an action or saying something that causes certain thoughts to be produced.

(50) (B) He will repeat that behavior.

Rewards are a popular concept to show acknowledgment and acceptance of certain behaviors. In this way, the individual will remember the reinforcement and likely repeat the action, as he thinks it is appropriate.

(51) (A) Professionals, parents and peers; the seriousness of the issue.

Behavior plans are created to reduce or limit certain types of behaviors or encourage others. These include various steps and procedures and are usually created by ABA professionals.

However, the severity of the behavior will determine who can create this plan for the client. In some cases, peers and parents can also do so.

(52) (D) Spontaneous recovery.

After an extinction burst, problematic behavior starts to increase. However, this can be controlled and sometimes starts to go away on its own without any reinforcement—known as spontaneous recovery.

In the question, when the dog stops associating the word with food, he stops obeying the command because it is now a different task.

(53) (B) Preventive strategy.

Understanding the reason for the occurrence of a specific behavior is a better way of decreasing it.

Preventive strategies are part of behavior plans that prevent inappropriate behaviors from occurring. These strategies avoid certain actions and plan to establish rules and guidelines.

(54) (D) Both (A) and (B).

There are many elements of a behavior plan that help limit undesirable behavior. This includes consequential strategies that control behavior and are essential to help professionals decide what will happen in case of inappropriate behavior.

Section 5: Documentation and Reporting

(55) (B) Lock all notes in a filing cabinet.

Any information about the client should be kept private. Family members should not be given access to it. Only concerned RBTs should have access to any paper documents that are not saved electronically. The best way to safeguard paper documents is to have them locked in a cabinet.

(56) (C) RBTs should keep in daily contact with their supervisors.

RBTs should communicate with their supervisor in an ongoing manner. To swiftly and amicably discuss concerns and problem areas, the RBT and supervisor must ensure receptive communication abilities.

(57) (D) Immediately inform her supervisor of her suspicions in accordance with the organization's rules.

An RBT must instantly inform her supervisor if she encounters suspicions of abuse. She should not wait, because it can jeopardize the client's life and mental health.

(58) (B) Ask the supervisory BCBA for additional training.

RBTs need to communicate with their supervisor as soon as possible if they feel they may not be able to do something.

(59) (B) The BCBA or supervisor will contact them to discuss their question.

RBTs are not allowed to discuss client details with stakeholders or the client's family. Only the supervisor or BCBA should discuss the appropriate details with stakeholders or the client's family.

(60) (D) All of the above.

Reporting entails writing session notes, communicating with the BCBA on a case and entering ABC data not included in the behavior intervention plan.

(61) (D) "The client banged his head repeatedly on the table for 30 seconds while making a loud 'aaa' sound. To curb the behavior, I set a pillow on the table. This was new behavior, according to the client's mother."

All conversations with supervisors should be objective. Additionally, it must be behavioral; specific behavior must be described while avoiding emotive or mentalistic language, such as "He became furious."

(62) (D) A certified behavior technician's behavior reduction plan is implemented mainly by the BCBA. To ensure expertise, he or she receives regular supervision from a qualified analyst.

Usually, under the direct supervision of a BCBA or BCaBA, the RBT's role in the service delivery system entails implementing measurement, evaluation, skill acquisition, behavior reduction, documenting and reporting, as well as maintaining professional conduct within the practice's limits.

(63) (A) Measurable, observable, objective.

The RBT creates operational definitions for certain behaviors after deciding they need to be measured. This is a more thorough definition of a behavior adapted to the particular client. MOO stands for measurable, observable and objective.

(64) (D) Both A and B.

A BCBA can practice independently and also be the supervisor of an RBT.

Section 6: Professional Conduct and Scope of Practice

(65) (B) BCBA-D, BCBA, BCaBA, RBT.

Credentials approved by the BCBA include BCBA-D, BCBA, BCaBA and RBT. An RBT is a high school credential of diploma level, BCBA is a master's degree and BCaBa is a bachelor's degree.

(66) (A) The RBT should comply with the feedback.

When a supervisor provides feedback, it is the RBT's responsibility to comply with it. The RBT should analyze the input and utilize it to improve performance.

(67) (C) Because it includes certification titles and examination content.

The misuse of confidential information, like examination content and certification titles, belonging to supervisors can lead to information breaches.

(68) (A) Family, caregivers and other professionals.

Stakeholders are the client's family, caregivers and other professionals. The supervisor, the RBT and the supervisor's family are not related to the client except in a professional manner.

(69) (D) Enhancing skills takes time and cannot be done immediately.

Supervisors must remember their job is to make RBTs become better technicians. They should also keep in mind that change comes slowly.

(70) (B) The client's family can analyze what can be done to help the client.

RBTs can involve the client's family to help the client improve behavior, and the family can also analyze what can make the client feel better.

(71) (A) It allows for an individualized perspective of supervisory notes.

Creating a system for documenting supervision experience is allowed for supervisors, according to the monthly BCBA experience standards. It makes it possible to have an individualized perspective on supervisory notes.

(72) (D) 5 percent.

Every RBT must obtain supervision for a minimum of 5 percent of the hours they spend offering services. The required amount of supervision is one hour. However, the BCBA encourages supervision of service delivery as much as possible.

(73) (D) It is necessary to evaluate insufficient client progress, poor performance and unethical behavior.

The RBT supervisor needs to describe strategies and outcomes regarding ineffective supervision, during which the supervisor will evaluate insufficient client progress, unsatisfactory performance and unethical behavior.

It is also important for the supervisor to monitor any unprofessional behavior shown by the RBT.

(74) (A) It can improve the RBT's performance.

The supervisor evaluates the RBT's strengths and weaknesses to help improve performance and set goals.

(75) (C) It allows them to understand the clients' problems and help deal with them.

Showing empathy toward a client is essential for RBTs. It can help them comprehend the client's problems and deal with them. So, RBTs need to reflect behavior that shows they care about human feelings and are not merely interested in the money offered.

Moreover, RBTs must be able to comprehend the client's issues and emotions. However, being excessively attached to the client is not advisable. Although RBTs should maintain a friendly relationship with the client, they should keep professional boundaries.

(76) (B) Specific behaviors observed, interventions used, and the client's response.

This approach aligns with ABA's emphasis on measurable and observable data to assess interventions' effectiveness and the client's progress. It provides a factual basis for making informed decisions about future treatment strategies.

(77) (B) Adherence to ethical guidelines and accurate data collection.

RBTs must follow ethical guidelines and accurately report data. Without these guidelines, all professional standards and treatment integrity would fall apart. The BCBA should focus on these to improve the quality of service.

(78) (C) Document the behavior and report it to the BCBA supervisor.

New behaviors could have significant clinical indications. Therefore, it is important to report them to the BCBA supervisor, who will ensure that the subsequent interventions are based on up-to-date and evidence-based science.

(79) (C) Accurate documentation of the client's behavior and the interventions used.

Accurate documentation is essential to evaluate the effectiveness of interventions and ensure continuity of care. It helps the RBT to understand the treatment plan and how to implement it.

(80) (B) Prepare a detailed report that includes the behavior, context, and any interventions attempted.

A detailed report will communicate all the necessary information to the RBT's supervisor. This will guarantee an effective plan that takes into consideration the nuances that are commonly missed by new RBTs.

(81) (B) Prepare a summary of recent client sessions.

A summary of recent client sessions improves service quality and creates a timeline with improvements and setbacks. This is one of the best ways to prepare for a supervised therapy session.

(82) (C) Demonstrate the intervention, observe the RBT's application, and provide feedback.

When a BCBA demonstrates the intervention and asks for feedback, the RBT swiftly develops important skills and ensures that interventions can be applied correctly. Ultimately, they hone all the necessary skills that an RBT should possess.

(83) (B) Accept the feedback and ask for clarification.

When an RBT accepts their supervisor's feedback, it promotes professional growth and understanding. RBTs should not forget that the entire purpose of supervision is to refine their skills and techniques.

(84) (B) Observe the RBT with a client at least once a month to provide direct feedback.

This requirement is essential for hands-on evaluation of the RBT's application of skills and interventions. Moreover, it facilitates tailored feedback and direct observation.

(85) (B) Communicate progress and challenges.

This behavior builds a positive supervisory relationship that prioritizes open communication and the willingness to learn from supervision. This is important for professional development.

Test 4

(1) A newly employed RBT attends her first session with a ten-year-old client diagnosed with autism spectrum disorder. She understands the importance of data collection in monitoring progress. What should her initial step be in the task analysis of data collection?

(A) Choose the most efficient data collection method.

(B) Determine the type of behavior to be observed.

(C) Gather necessary materials (e.g., pen, paper, timer).

(D) Eliminate any potential distractions in the environment.

(2) An RBT observes a client to record the frequency of a specific behavior to assess its occurrence compared to the average. However, he realizes the environment is noisy, which could affect the reliability of the collected data. What should the RBT do first to ensure accurate data collection?

(A) Start data collection immediately so as not to miss any behavior.

(B) Move the client to a quieter environment.

(C) Continue the observation and note the noisy environment as a variable.

(D) Ask for assistance to control the noise level.

(3) An RBT is about to collect data about a client's behavior but realizes she does not have a standard form to record their identifying information. What is the most appropriate next step for her to take in this situation?

(A) Proceed with the observation and try to memorize the client's details.

(B) Use a notebook to write down the client's identifying information.

(C) Postpone the data collection until a standard form is available.

(D) Collect data without recording the client's identifying information.

(4) During a session, an RBT notices a new behavior in the client that was not previously observed. What should they do in this scenario?

(A) Immediately inform the client's family about the new behavior.

(B) Record the frequency and context of the new behavior to analyze its impact.

(C) Ignore the new behavior and focus only on the predefined data collection.

(D) Advise the client to stop the new behavior.

(5) An RBT needs to decide between continuous and discontinuous measurements for a client who exhibits a behavior with varying intensity and duration. What factor should be the most critical in their decision-making process?

(A) Client's comfort.

(B) Data accuracy and relevance.

(C) Time.

(D) Ease of set up.

(6) During a data collection session, an RBT realizes that the client's behavior is influenced by the presence of certain stimuli in the environment. What should be the RBT's immediate course of action to ensure the integrity of the data collection process?

(A) Ignore the stimuli as they are part of the natural environment.

(B) Identify and possibly remove the stimuli to control extraneous variables.

(C) Note the stimuli as an observation but continue as planned.

(D) Change the focus of the session to the stimuli instead of the client's behavior.

(7) An RBT conducts a task analysis and has gathered all necessary materials. They are about to observe a client but notice the room is quite cluttered and busy. How should they proceed to ensure a reliable data collection process?

(A) Start the observation and note the environment's condition.

(B) Reschedule the session to a more controlled environment.

(C) Organize and declutter the room before starting.

(D) Continue as planned and assume the clutter will not affect the data.

(8) An RBT needs to choose a data collection method for behavior that occurs at a high frequency. What should be their main consideration in the selection of the most suitable method?

(A) Uses the least amount of time.

(B) Allows for the most detailed notes.

(C) Is the least intrusive to the client.

(D) Provides the most accurate representation of the behavior.

(9) During a data collection session, an RBT realizes that the chosen method does not accurately capture the client's behavior due to its complexity. What is the most appropriate action for the RBT to take in this scenario?

(A) Continue with the chosen method for consistency.

(B) Modify the current method to capture the behavior's complexity more precisely.

(C) Immediately stop the session and consult with a supervisor.

(D) Switch to a more suitable data collection method if possible.

(10) An RBT collects data on a new client and notices several previously unreported behaviors. They need to ensure these behaviors are accurately recorded for future analysis. What should be the main focus?

(A) The frequency and intensity of the new behaviors.

(B) Possible triggers and consequences of the new behaviors.

(C) Time of day and setting in which the new behaviors occur.

(D) The client's mood and physical condition when the new behaviors occur.

(11) An RBT observes a client in a classroom and needs to collect data discreetly. The client's behavior is sporadic and unpredictable. Which data collection method should the RBT prioritize in this context?

(A) A continuous recording.

(B) Samples from certain times or situations.

(C) Extensive setup and materials.

(D) A method that involves the teacher's input during the session.

(12) After completing a data collection session, an RBT realizes that some data may be inaccurate due to unexpected environmental variables. What should be the next best step to maintain the integrity of the data collected?

(A) Discard the entire session's data and plan a new session.

(B) Analyze the data but note the potential inaccuracies due to environmental variables.

(C) Report the issue to a supervisor and seek guidance on how to proceed.

(D) Ignore the discrepancies and use the data as if it were accurate.

(13) An RBT is instructed to use digital forms for data collection but is more comfortable with paper forms. If they consider the importance of accurate and efficient data collection, what should be the approach?

(A) Stick to paper forms since it is their comfort zone.

(B) Transition to digital forms and seek training if necessary.

(C) Use both paper and digital forms to ensure data is captured accurately.

(D) Avoid data collection until they are fully comfortable with digital forms.

(14) An RBT conducts a session that focuses on a specific behavior but notices that the client exhibits another significant behavior. What should the RBT's approach be in this situation?

(A) Focus only on the specific behavior as initially planned.

(B) Record the new behavior and analyze its relation to the specific behavior.

(C) Immediately stop the session and consult with a supervisor.

(D) Ignore the new behavior as it is not part of the session's goal.

(15) An RBT conducts a preference assessment to identify potential reinforcers for a new skill acquisition program. They have an array of toys and food items. Which assessment method should they use to identify the most preferred item?

(A) Multiple stimulus with replacement.

(B) Multiple stimulus without replacement.

(C) Paired stimulus.

(D) Single stimulus.

(16) During a preference assessment, an RBT notices that the client takes a significantly longer time to choose between items. What does this observation indicate in the context of a multiple stimulus without replacement assessment?

(A) The client does not understand the assessment.

(B) The client has equal preference for the items.

(C) The behavior of the client is interfering with the assessment.

(D) The time taken indicates the client's least and most preferred items.

(17) An RBT wants to conduct a preference assessment for a client who shows problematic behavior when preferred items are removed. Which assessment method is best suited for this client?

(A) Multiple stimulus with replacement.

(B) Multiple stimulus without replacement.

(C) Paired stimulus.

(D) Single stimulus.

(18) An RBT conducts a preference assessment in a classroom where the client can freely choose among various items or activities. Which method should the RBT use to observe the client's selections and interactions with the items over time?

(A) Multiple stimulus with replacement.

(B) Multiple stimulus without replacement.

(C) Paired stimulus.

(D) Free-operant observations.

(19) During a preference assessment, an RBT pairs a highly preferred item with a low-preferred item. The client consistently chooses the highly preferred item. Which type of preference assessment is used?

(A) Multiple stimulus with replacement.

(B) Multiple stimulus without replacement.

(C) Paired stimulus.

(D) Single stimulus.

(20) An RBT wants to quickly identify a hierarchy of preferred items for a client who does not show problematic behavior when a preferred toy is taken away. Which method should the RBT use for the most accurate and efficient results?

(A) Multiple stimulus with replacement.

(B) Multiple stimulus without replacement.

(C) Paired stimulus.

(D) Single stimulus.

(21) In order to determine the preferred reinforcers to use for a client's appropriate behavior, which method should the RBT use first to gather information about the client's preferences?

(A) Free-operant observations assessment.

(B) Single stimulus assessment.

(C) Open-ended questions or a multiple-choice format.

(D) Multiple stimulus with replacement assessment.

(22) A client can choose preferred items from an array of choices. However, they display problematic behavior when the item is removed. The RBT wants to identify the most preferred items but keep all options available to the client. Which preference assessment method should be used?

(A) Multiple stimulus with replacement.

(B) Multiple stimulus without replacement.

(C) Paired stimulus.

(D) Free-operant observations.

(23) A client experiences difficulties when he tries to choose between highly preferred and low-preferred items. Which method is most appropriate for this client to avoid frustration and ensure accurate assessment results?

(A) Multiple stimulus with replacement.

(B) Multiple stimulus without replacement.

(C) Paired stimulus.

(D) Single stimulus.

(24) An RBT noticed the patient's preferences during an assessment. It was clear that the patient chose a specific toy repeatedly over several sessions. What does this behavior indicate about the toy?

(A) It is a potential distraction in the assessment.

(B) It is a potential reinforcer for the client.

(C) It is not suitable for further sessions.

(D) It is only suitable for free-operant observations.

(25) A non-verbal client shows an interest in certain toys but does not demonstrate clear choices when multiple options are presented. Which preference assessment method should the RBT consider to accommodate the client's needs?

(A) Multiple stimulus with replacement.

(B) Multiple stimulus without replacement.

(C) Paired stimulus.

(D) Single stimulus.

(26) In a classroom, a twelve-year-old boy freely interacts with different items. The RBT records the items the client interacts with the most. What is this type of assessment?

(A) Multiple stimulus with replacement.

(B) Multiple stimulus without replacement.

(C) Paired stimulus.

(D) Free-operant observations.

(27) An RBT attempts to identify reinforcers that decrease a client's inappropriate behavior. The client tends to scream when dissatisfied. Which of these criteria should be used to select reinforcers for the client?

(A) Most preferred items in the assessment.

(B) Least preferred items to avoid overstimulation.

(C) Items that have not been selected during the assessment.

(D) Items that were selected by the client's parents or caregivers.

(28) An eight-year-old female presents with her parents, who complain of her difficult behavior. The RBT tries to reinforce patience in the client. They decide to use a preference assessment to select suitable stimuli. What is the main goal of this assessment?

(A) Punish the inappropriate behavior.

(B) Reward the client for showing patience.

(C) Identify stimuli that can motivate positive behavior.

(D) Teach the client to select items quickly.

(29) In a multiple stimulus without replacement assessment, an RBT observes that a client selects a particular item first. What is the interpretation of this action?

(A) Neutral preference of the client.

(B) Most preferred item of the client.

(C) Least preferred item of the client.

(D) Requires replacement with a more preferred item.

(30) An RBT is required to formulate a written skill acquisition plan for a client with developmental disabilities. They had already conducted a task analysis and broken down the skill into smaller steps. What is the next immediate step to prepare the plan according to the essential components?

(A) Select an appropriate reinforcement schedule.

(B) Identify the individual's current level of functioning.

(C) Create a detailed schedule of when each step will be taught.

(D) Review the information and situation regularly.

(31) A behavior analyst works on a skill acquisition plan that teaches a new skill. To ensure the plan's effectiveness, what component must be included to measure the actual behavior change?

(A) A generalization and maintenance plan.

(B) Accurate measurement of the target behavior.

(C) A plan for reinforcement.

(D) A detailed description of the steps.

(32) A middle school student's progress in skill acquisition has stagnated for several months. To understand the cause and make necessary adjustments, what type of data should be the RBT's focus?

(A) Frequency data.

(B) Duration data.

(C) Partial interval data.

(D) Scatterplot data.

(33) During class, an RBT learns about the importance of a clear mastery criterion. What is the main purpose of a mastery criterion in the skill acquisition plan?

(A) Determine when the client has sufficiently learned the skill.

(B) Establish a reinforcement schedule.

(C) Decide the prompting strategies to be used.

(D) Outline the consequences for correct and incorrect responses.

(34) A behavior analyst wants to ensure that a learned skill is maintained over time. Which component should be included in the plan to address this need?

(A) Description of the target skill being taught.

(B) Generalization and maintenance plan.

(C) Specific objective that shows the development of a skill.

(D) Reactionary techniques for unwanted behaviors.

(35) During a session, the RBT is tasked to teach a new skill to a client with a written skill acquisition plan. The client does not respond well to the current strategy. What is the most appropriate next step?

(A) Change the prompting strategies to promote student independence.

(B) Focus on reinforcers to correct responses more frequently.

(C) Continue with the current strategy for consistency.

(D) Implement reactionary techniques for unwanted behaviors.

(36) An RBT is tasked to craft a skill acquisition plan and ensure the client is motivated to learn the new skill. Which of the following components should be included in the plan?

(A) A description of the target skill.

(B) The required educational materials.

(C) An appropriate reinforcement schedule.

(D) The consequences of correct or incorrect responses.

(37) During a skill acquisition session, an RBT observes that a client performs the target behavior correctly after specific prompts. To assess the effectiveness of the instructional methods, what type of data should the RBT mainly collect?

(A) Frequency data.

(B) Duration data.

(C) Partial interval data.

(D) Permanent product data.

(38) An analyst formulates a written skill acquisition plan. Which element must be defined to evaluate if an activity or goal successfully teaches the desired skills?

(A) A specific objective that shows the development of a skill.

(B) The prompting strategies to be used.

(C) The consequences for correct or incorrect responses.

(D) Reinforcement techniques.

(39) An RBT works with a client who occasionally displays unwanted behavior during skill acquisition sessions. What component should be included in the skill acquisition plan to address this issue effectively?

(A) Generalization and maintenance plan.

(B) Reactionary techniques for unwanted conduct or delayed skill display.

(C) Detailed description of the steps.

(D) Methods to regularly review the information and situation.

(40) A client requires instructions to write. This approach follows a skill acquisition plan. He makes a mistake when writing a letter. According to the essential components of a written skill acquisition plan, what should the RBT's immediate response be?

(A) Ignore the mistake and continue with the session.

(B) Use error correction techniques to address the mistake.

(C) Reinforce the client since they attempted the task.

(D) Change the teaching material.

(41) An RBT is in the midst of data collection on a client's skill acquisition progress. They notice a pattern in the client's behavior that seems related to the time of day. What type of data collection method is likely being used here?

(A) Frequency data.

(B) Duration data.

(C) Partial interval data.

(D) Scatterplot data.

(42) A behavior analyst plans to fade service hours but maintain the therapeutic potential after a client has reached their skill goals. Which component of the skill acquisition plan addresses this process?

(A) Presentation methods.

(B) Strategies for skill upkeep and service termination.

(C) Instructions for desired responses.

(D) SR +/- reinforcement and plan for reinforcement.

(43) An RBT analyzes data from skill acquisition sessions to predict how the client will behave in certain situations. This predictive analysis is particularly helpful for what application of behavioral data?

(A) Market research.

(B) Government policymaking.

(C) Mental health treatment development.

(D) Instructional method effectiveness.

(44) As part of their training, an RBT must implement a written skill acquisition plan and gather data to assess the program's effectiveness. Which of these is an essential part of the plan that allows for this data-driven approach?

(A) Techniques to gather and display data.

(B) A detailed plan of when each task step will be taught.

(C) A specific objective that shows the development of a skill.

(D) SR +/- reinforcement and plan for reinforcement.

(45) An RBT works with a child who has difficulty in the transition between activities. They implement a visual timer to help the child understand the time left to complete a task. What is the main benefit of a visual timer in this scenario?

(A) Provide a strict schedule for the child to follow.

(B) Help the child mentally prepare for the transition.

(C) Act as a disciplinary tool.

(D) Eliminate the need for verbal reminders from the RBT.

(46) An RBT notices that a seven-year-old girl exhibits escapist behavior during a teeth-brushing routine. The RBT wants to reduce this behavior through the introduction of replacement behavior. Which option best aligns with ABA principles to choose an appropriate replacement behavior?

(A) Teach the client to scream less loudly to express discomfort.

(B) Allow the child to skip teeth brushing whenever they show escapist behavior.

(C) Introduce a fun song related to teeth brushing to make the routine more enjoyable.

(D) Ignore the escapist behavior to discourage it.

(47) The parents of a child complain that their son bangs items on the table to gain attention. The RBT is tasked to create a behavior reduction plan. What component is vital to include in this plan?

(A) A detailed description of the child's favorite activities.

(B) A clear consequence strategy for inappropriate behavior.

(C) An award system for every task completed by the child.

(D) A list of the child's dislikes and likes.

(48) A client with autism shows signs of stress when he transitions between tasks. The RBT decides to introduce coping strategies. Which coping strategy aligns with ABA practices to assist the client and keep them calm?

(A) Encourage the client to express stress through physical outbursts.

(B) Avoid transitions altogether to prevent stress.

(C) Increase the speed of transitions to reduce stress.

(D) Implement deep breathing exercises before transitions.

(49) To work on the transition strategies of a client, the RBT uses photos as visual cues to indicate the next task. What is the main benefit of using visual objects as transition strategies?

(A) Deliver a punishment for inappropriate behavior.

(B) Provide a strict and inflexible transition routine.

(C) Increase the probability of displaying the demanded behavior and decrease challenging behavior.

(D) Eliminate the need for the RBT's involvement in the process.

(50) During an ABA session, the RBT identifies that a client's behavior is problematic when she snatches things from others. They plan to introduce a replacement behavior. What is a key consideration before choosing a replacement behavior?

(A) It should be more complex than the original behavior.

(B) It fulfills the same purpose as the client's original behavior.

(C) It takes longer to perform than the original behavior.

(D) It is less socially acceptable than the original behavior.

(51) A session is scheduled to teach a client how to request attention appropriately. What is the purpose of this replacement behavior?

(A) Make the client's behavior more complex.

(B) Eliminate all forms of bad communication from the client.

(C) Increase the frequency of the client's behavior for attention.

(D) Provide a faster and easier alternative.

(52) An RBT prepares a behavior reduction plan for a client. What is an important component that should be included to ensure the plan's effectiveness?

(A) A detailed plan for the RBT's vacation days.

(B) A list of the client's favorite movies and books.

(C) Data collection procedures to observe and measure the target behavior.

(D) A strict schedule for the client to follow.

(53) A mother complains that her child commonly runs away from the table when it is time to do homework. The RBT understands this as an *escape* function of behavior. What is an appropriate replacement behavior to teach?

(A) Run to a different room but do the homework.

(B) Wait for the child to do the homework by themselves.

(C) Teach the child to request a break after a certain period of work.

(D) Remove homework from the child's routine entirely.

(54) An RBT uses a behavior reduction plan to manage the aggressive behavior of a ten-year-old child. The parents are involved in the plan. What role should the parents play in this behavior reduction plan?

(A) Strictly enforce the consequences at home.

(B) Provide constant rewards for the child.

(C) Understand and support the components of the plan.

(D) Take over the plan entirely over time.

(55) The parents of a three-year-old boy state that other parents complained that their child frequently grabs the toys of other children, which makes them cry. An RBT is tasked with this child's behavior education. What is a key attribute of this replacement behavior?

(A) Equally forceful but in a different form.

(B) Consumes more time than the original behavior.

(C) Socially acceptable and easier than the original behavior.

(D) Slow and flexible to avoid child abuse.

(56) An RBT must implement transition strategies for a twelve-year-old boy with autism who struggles with changes in routine. What type of transition strategy could be most beneficial for this client?

(A) Enforce rapid transitions.

(B) Use a visual timer to provide a clear indication of time left for a task.

(C) Remove all transitions from the client's routine.

(D) Encourage abrupt changes to enhance the client's adaptability.

(57) An RBT needs to create a transition strategy for a client who responds well to visual cues. They want to make the transition between activities smoother. Which strategy should the RBT consider?

(A) Implement a visual timer or use photo icons.

(B) Use complex verbal instructions for transitions.

(C) Make sudden changes without any cues.

(D) Increase the duration of activities to avoid transitions.

(58) An RBT works to reduce a child's problematic behavior. The client's behavior can be very severe. Who is best equipped to write and oversee this behavior reduction plan?

(A) The client's parents.

(B) An RBT with minimal experience in behavior plans.

(C) A professional at the BCBA or BCaBA level.

(D) Any individual unrelated to the ABA therapy process.

(59) An RBT teaches a client about the function of behavior and how it accesses tangibles. The parents say that their child commonly takes toys without permission. What would be an effective replacement behavior to teach the client?

(A) Encourage the client to take toys more discreetly.

(B) Reward the client each time they take a toy.

(C) Remove all toys from the client's environment.

(D) Teach the client to ask politely for the toys.

(60) For the first time since graduation, an RBT receives supervision. The supervisor explains the purpose and goals of the supervision. According to the Supervisor Curriculum Training Outline, what is the benefit of a purpose and goal statement?

(A) Helps the RBT understand the punitive measures for non-compliance.

(B) Creates the context for clear communication and ensures procedural fidelity.

(C) Allows the supervisor to exercise authority over the RBT.

(D) Provides an opportunity for the supervisor to showcase their skills.

(61) During a supervision session, the supervisor notices that the RBT's client does not progress as expected. What should the supervisor's immediate next step be?

(A) Identify and discuss the causes of insufficient client progress, poor performance, or unethical behavior.

(B) Terminate the RBT for poor performance.

(C) Increase the frequency of supervision to daily sessions.

(D) Change the client's treatment plan.

(62) A new supervisor plans to take on several RBTs for supervision. According to the Supervisor Curriculum Training Outline, what must the supervisor consider before they establish the supervisory relationship?

(A) The supervisor's personal preference for clients.

(B) Feasible supervision capacity based on available time and resources.

(C) Financial benefits of multiple RBT supervision.

(D) Reputation of the RBTs in the field.

(63) An RBT supervisor develops a structured plan to supervise an RBT. What is a key component that must be included in this plan?

(A) A detailed biography of the RBT.

(B) A strict disciplinary action plan for any mistakes made by the RBT.

(C) Supervision content and evaluation of competence for the RBT.

(D) A comprehensive list of all the clients the RBT will serve.

(64) A supervisor documents their supervision experience with an RBT. According to the BCBA experience standards, what flexibility is allowed in the documentation process?

(A) An informal verbal agreement instead of written documentation

(B) The supervisor can personally develop a system to document the supervision experience.

(C) Good performance by the RBT warrants the discontinuation of documentation.

(D) The supervisor can delegate the responsibility of documentation to the RBT.

(65) An RBT is scheduled to be observed by their supervisor during a session with a thirteen-year-old child with autism. According to the monthly BCBA experience standards, what is the minimum requirement for such observations?

(A) Monthly.

(B) Weekly.

(C) Every six months.

(D) At the supervisor's discretion.

(66) A supervisor instructs an RBT on how to improve their service delivery. What is the first step the supervisor should take based on the four-step supervision process?

(A) Demonstrate how the problem can be solved.

(B) Observe the RBT when they perform the particular task.

(C) Provide feedback in the form of notes.

(D) Instruct the RBT based on what the supervisor notices.

(67) During the past six months, an RBT worked on their skills after receiving feedback from an RBT supervisor. How can the supervisor motivate them if they show progress?

(A) Set goals and provide feedback once the goals have been met.

(B) Ensure that their skills rapidly improve to reach the next level.

(C) Provide financial incentives for every improvement noted.

(D) Compare the RBT's performance with other RBTs to build a sense of competition.

(68) An RBT is part of a tiered service delivery model under the direction of a BCBA. What is the role of the RBT in this model?

(A) Develop treatment plans and provide clinical recommendations.

(B) Implement the service plans for the client and assist the advisory team.

(C) Supervise other RBTs and BCaBAs.

(D) Handle all the administrative tasks for the BCBA.

(69) A supervisor provides constructive feedback to an RBT about their performance. According to professional conduct standards, how should the RBT respond to this feedback?

(A) Disregard the feedback if it does not align with their perspective.

(B) Comply with the feedback and work on their weak points.

(C) Report the supervisor for harassment if the feedback is redundant.

(D) Only accept positive feedback.

(70) An RBT faces legal charges and is under investigation by their employer. According to professional conduct standards, what is the RBT required to do?

(A) Keep the information confidential and not report it.

(B) Self-report the situation within thirty days once aware of it.

(C) Wait for the employer to take the first step.

(D) Only report if found guilty.

(71) An RBT supervisor explains to an RBT the importance of supervision. What reason should the supervisor highlight as a key purpose of supervision?

(A) Ensure that the RBT feels constantly monitored.

(B) Create a hierarchy to maintain order.

(C) Provide high-quality services that result in client improvement.

(D) Confirm that the RBT has completed documentation and paperwork.

(72) An RBT supervisor discusses strategies with the RBT for a client who shows insufficient progress. What should the focus of the discussion be?

(A) Explore the potential reasons for insufficient client progress.

(B) Assign blame for the client's lack of progress.

(C) Hope the client's progress improves in the upcoming sessions.

(D) Replace the RBT with a more experienced one.

(73) During preparation for a supervision session, an RBT supervisor plans to review the RBT's performance and provide feedback. What aspect of the supervision plan ensures the effectiveness of this session?

(A) Focus on the RBT's weaknesses.

(B) Prioritize administrative tasks over observational feedback.

(C) Make the session as detailed as possible.

(D) Develop a structured plan that contains supervision content and an evaluation of the RBT's competence.

(74) During a supervision session, an RBT expresses concerns about their workload and client interactions. What approach should the supervisor take to address these concerns effectively?

(A) Dismiss the RBT's concerns as irrelevant.

(B) Explore feasible solutions based on available resources.

(C) Instruct the RBT to manage their time better.

(D) Explain to the RBT that a heavy workload is important to boost adaptability.

(75) A supervisor observes an RBT's session with a client and plans to provide feedback. What is the supervisor's next immediate step after the demonstration?

(A) Take a break and postpone the feedback to the next session.

(B) Observe the RBT as they perform the task and keep in mind the previous problems.

(C) Promote or demote the RBT based on their demonstration.

(D) Provide feedback if the RBT requests it.

(76) An RBT has completed 100 hours of work in a month. According to the supervision requirements, how many hours of supervision should the RBT receive for that month?

(A) At least five hours.

(B) Ten hours.

(C) Fifteen hours.

(D) Twenty hours.

(77) A BCBA supervisor plans the structure of supervision for an RBT. According to the requirements, how should the supervisor ensure effective supervision?

(A) Hold at least two monthly real-time face-to-face meetings.

(B) Supervise the RBT through online platforms.

(C) Have daily in-person meetings with the RBT.

(D) Conduct group sessions.

(78) An RBT struggles with a specific aspect of their role and needs guidance. How should the supervisor provide direction to the RBT?

(A) Give feedback during annual evaluations.

(B) Communicate clear and timely feedback during supervision sessions.

(C) Instruct the RBT to figure it out on their own.

(D) Delegate the responsibility for feedback to another competent RBT.

(79) During a supervision session, the BCBA supervisor observes that the RBT does not implement ABA techniques properly. What should be the supervisor's first step according to the supervision process?

(A) Terminate the RBT's contract.

(B) Ignore this issue since guidelines and techniques are not always helpful.

(C) Provide instruction on the correct implementation of ABA techniques.

(D) Report the RBT to the licensing board for malpractice.

(80) An RBT is scheduled for a supervision session with their BCBA supervisor. What is the main role of the RBT to ensure effective communication during this session?

(A) Understand the supervisor's feedback and ask questions.

(B) Dictate the session's agenda based on their preferences.

(C) Challenge the supervisor's feedback when it seems impractical.

(D) Avoid discussion with the supervisor to prevent penalties.

(81) A BCBA supervisor needs to observe an RBT who provides services for a child with difficult behavior. What is the minimum observation frequency?

(A) Once a week.

(B) Once a month.

(C) Once every six months.

(D) Annually.

(82) An RBT supervisor identifies a problem in the RBT's service delivery. After instructing the RBT on improvements, what is the supervisor's next step?

(A) Demonstrate how the problem can be solved.

(B) Wait for the RBT to request further clarification.

(C) Move on to another topic.

(D) Leave the RBT to practice on their own.

(83) An RBT faces a situation that requires rapid attention. According to effective communication guidelines, what should the RBT do?

(A) Wait for the next scheduled supervision session to discuss the issue.

(B) Contact the supervisor immediately to address the urgent matter.

(C) Try to solve the problem independently.

(D) Discuss the issue with colleagues.

(84) An RBT receives feedback from their supervisor during a supervision session. How should the RBT respond to this feedback professionally?

(A) Accept the feedback and work on areas of improvement.

(B) Disregard the feedback if it conflicts with the RBT's previous education.

(C) Prove why the supervisor's feedback might be biased.

(D) Report the supervisor if the feedback is too harsh.

(85) A child's case requires a specific amount of supervision hours according to the RBT's assessment. However, the authorized hours for supervision may need adjustment throughout the treatment. What does this imply about the supervision process?

(A) Supervision hours are fixed and cannot be changed once determined.

(B) Supervision hours are irrelevant and do not impact the client's treatment.

(C) Supervision hours should always be minimized to reduce costs.

(D) Authorized supervision hours are just general parameters and may be adjusted based on the client's needs.

Test 4 Answers and Explanations

(1) (B) Determine the type of behavior to be observed.

The initial step in task analysis of data collection is to determine the type of behavior to be observed. Different behaviors require different measurement strategies to achieve the most valid results. Understanding the behavior type before an RBT chooses methods or gathers materials is fundamental as it guides the entire data collection process.

(2) (D) Ask for assistance to control the noise level.

Environment control to eliminate distractions is vital for accurate data collection. A noisy room can affect the reliability of the data. Before an RBT proceeds to data collection, it is essential to address these environmental factors to ensure that the data accurately reflects the client's behavior.

(3) (B) Use a notebook to write down the client's identifying information.

When standard forms are unavailable, an RBT should accurately record the client's identifying information for future reference and analysis. A notebook ensures that essential details (e.g., name, date of birth, specifics of the observed behavior) are not missed, which maintains the integrity of the data collection process.

(4) (B) Record the frequency and context of the new behavior to analyze its impact.

When an RBT observes and records new behaviors, it provides valuable insights into the client's progress and the therapy's effectiveness. They should document the frequency and context of the new behavior to analyze its impact and relevance to the client's treatment plan.

(5) (B) Data accuracy and relevance.

The choice between continuous and discontinuous measurements should be based on the accuracy and relevance of the data each method provides. It is important to select a method that accurately captures the behavior's intensity and duration.

(6) (B) Identify and possibly remove the stimuli to control extraneous variables.

An RBT should identify and remove stimuli that influence the client's behavior to ensure the data's integrity. The minimization of variables increases the accuracy of behavior assessment and produces more reliable and valid data.

(7) (C) Organize and declutter the room before starting.

A controlled environment free of distractions is vital for accurate data collection. Room organization is part of this process to improve the quality of the data and ensure that it truly reflects the client's behavior.

(8) (D) Provides the most accurate representation of the behavior.

When an RBT chooses a data collection method for high-frequency behaviors, the priority should be to select a method that most accurately represents the behavior. Accurately capturing the nuances and frequency of the behavior is indispensable for valid analysis and the development of an effective treatment plan.

(9) (D) Switch to a more suitable data collection method if possible.

If the chosen data collection method does not accurately capture the complexity of the client's behavior, it is essential to switch to a more suitable method. RBTs must accurately collect data to understand the behavior and formulate an effective intervention strategy.

(10) (B) Possible triggers and consequences of the new behaviors.

RBTs should focus on possible triggers and consequences when new behaviors occur. This approach allows them to understand the behaviors in context, which makes it easier to create a comprehensive analysis that can inform future treatment strategies and adjustments to the intervention plan.

(11) (B) Samples from certain times or situations.

In a classroom where the behavior is sporadic, and the RBT needs to be discreet, a data collection method that samples certain times or situations is ideal. This approach allows for focused data collection and ensures that the natural setting is not disrupted.

(12) (B) Analyze the data but note the potential inaccuracies due to environmental variables.

When faced with unexpected environmental variables, RBTs must first analyze the collected data and note potential inaccuracies. Next, they need to acknowledge these variables to ensure a transparent and comprehensive analysis, which allows for adjustments in future data collection sessions and treatment planning.

(13) (B) Transition to digital forms and seek training if necessary.

Adapting digital forms for data collection boosts efficiency and accuracy. Although many RBTs still prefer paper forms, digital forms provide many benefits. This is why it is important to integrate digital forms in training courses to ensure that new graduates are more comfortable with this technology.

(14) (B) Record the new behavior and analyze its relation to the specific behavior.

When a significant new behavior is observed, it is important to record and analyze its relation to the specific behavior under observation. This comprehensive approach ensures that all relevant data is captured and provides a holistic view of the client's behavior to facilitate informed treatment decisions.

(15) (A) Multiple stimulus with replacement.

The multiple stimulus with replacement assessment is suitable when the RBT aims to identify the most preferred item. It allows a child to choose from an array of items and replace the chosen one each time. This method maintains a constant number of choices and replaces selected items with new stimuli. Eventually, it will help to determine the client's most preferred items through repeated selection.

(16) (D) The time taken indicates the client's least and most preferred items.

In a multiple stimulus without replacement assessment, the client's decision-making duration indicates their preference levels for the items. Longer decision times suggest uncertainty or lower preference. Conversely, quicker choices usually indicate higher preference. This timing is critical to understanding the client's preferences and arranging them from most to least preferred.

(17) (D) Single stimulus.

The single stimulus assessment is most appropriate for clients with challenging behavior when preferred items are removed. The client can engage with preferred items until they stop or show disinterest. This method avoids the removal of items, which prevents possible unwanted behaviors associated with item removal.

(18) (D) Free-operant observations.

Free-operant observations are most suitable in a classroom where the client can freely choose among various items or activities. This method allows the RBT to observe the client's spontaneous interactions with different items over time. As a result, the RBT is provided with insight into the client's natural preferences without the constraints of structured choice-making.

(19) (C) Paired stimulus.

The paired stimulus preference assessment presents two items simultaneously. After that, the client can choose between a highly preferred item and a low-preferred item. The consistent choice of the highly preferred item over the other indicates the client's preference, which makes the paired stimulus method suitable for this scenario.

(20) (B) Multiple stimulus without replacement.

The multiple stimulus without replacement assessment is quick and accurate for children who do not engage in problematic behavior when a preferred toy is taken away. It allows the client to choose preferred items one by one without the need to replace them. Ultimately, this establishes a preference hierarchy from most to least preferred.

(21) (C) Open-ended questions or a multiple-choice format.

Before an RBT starts a formal preference assessment, it is beneficial to gather preliminary information about the client's preferences through open-ended questions or a multiple-choice format. This approach involves the parents, caregivers, and teachers to provide a broader perspective on the client's preferences.

(22) (A) Multiple stimulus with replacement.

The multiple stimulus with replacement assessment is ideal for clients who demonstrate problematic behavior if a preferred item is removed. This method allows clients to select their most preferred items while keeping all options available. The difference between this approach and multiple stimulus without replacement is that the former encourages item replacement.

(23) (D) Single stimulus.

The single stimulus assessment is most appropriate for clients with challenging behavior when preferred items are removed. It allows the client to engage with preferred items until they stop or show disinterest. This method avoids the removal of items, which prevents possible unwanted behaviors associated with item removal.

(24) (B) It is a potential reinforcer for the client.

Consistent selection of a specific toy over several sessions in a preference assessment suggests that the client highly prefers the item. Therefore, it could be a potent reinforcer, which makes it a valuable tool for motivating and reinforcing desired behaviors.

(25) (D) Single stimulus.

The single stimulus assessment is suitable for non-verbal clients or those who show interest but do not make clear choices among multiple options. The presentation of one item at a time allows the client to interact with each item without the pressure or confusion of multiple choices.

(26) (D) Free-operant observations.

Free-operant observations study the client while they interact with various items or activities freely. There are no structured prompts or limitations. The documentation of the items that the client interacts with the most provides valuable insights into their natural preferences and can be especially informative in a classroom setting where the client has access to many choices.

(27) (A) Most preferred items in the assessment.

Preference assessments aim to identify the most preferred items that can act as potential reinforcers. When used effectively, these preferred items can help reduce inappropriate behaviors, such as screaming. The therapist uses the preferred items as positive reinforcement for alternative and appropriate behaviors.

(28) (C) Identify stimuli that can motivate positive behavior.

Preference assessments are conducted to determine what will act as a motivation for the client and at what specific point in time. The main goal is to identify stimuli that can act as reinforcers, which boosts the chances of positive behavior in the future.

(29) (B) Most preferred item of the client.

In a multiple stimulus without replacement assessment, the client's initial selection indicates their most preferred item. This preference is shown when the client chooses that particular item first among the array of choices.

(30) (C) Create a detailed schedule of when each step will be taught.

After the RBT conducts a task analysis and breaks the skill into smaller steps, the next immediate step in a skill acquisition plan is to create a detailed schedule. This schedule outlines when each task step will be taught, which provides a structured framework for the instruction process. It ensures that each component of the skill is taught in a systematic and organized manner.

(31) (B) Accurate measurement of the target behavior.

An important component of a skill acquisition plan is the accurate measurement of the target behavior. This measurement allows behavior analysts to assess the progress and effectiveness of the intervention. Based on the quantification of the client's performance, RBTs can determine if the client improves, stagnates, or worsens.

(32) (A) Frequency data.

When a student's progress has stagnated, it is critical to focus on frequency data. This data type provides information on how often a behavior occurs within a given timeframe. Therefore, it provides insights into a student's learning patterns and the effectiveness of the instructional methods. The analysis of this data helps RBTs understand the client's pace and identify areas of improvement.

(33) (A) Determine when the client has sufficiently learned the skill.

A mastery criterion is included in the skill acquisition plan to determine when the client has sufficiently learned the skill. This criterion sets a clear standard for performance, which allows RBTs to measure when a client has achieved the desired level of proficiency.

(34) (B) Generalization and maintenance plan.

It is essential to include a generalization and maintenance plan in the skill acquisition approach to ensure that the skill is maintained over time. This component outlines strategies that confirm the client can apply the learned skills in various contexts and retain them over time.

(35) (A) Change the prompting strategies to promote student independence.

If the client does not respond well to the current prompting strategy, the immediate action, according to the plan's components, would be to change it to promote student independence. This adjustment is important to adapt to the client's learning style and needs.

(36) (C) An appropriate reinforcement schedule.

An appropriate reinforcement schedule in the skill acquisition plan is vital to motivate the client to learn a new skill. Reinforcement schedules specify how and when the reinforcements are delivered, which makes the learning process effective.

(37) (A) Frequency data.

To assess the effectiveness of the instructional methods, the RBT should mainly focus on frequency data collection. This data type provides insights into how frequently the target behavior occurs. This allows the RBT to assess the success of the prompting strategy and the client's responsiveness to the teaching approach. It also helps evaluate the immediate impact of the instructional methods on the client's learning process.

(38) (A) A specific objective that shows the development of a skill.

A key element in a written skill acquisition plan is to define a specific objective that shows the development of a skill. This clear goal setting allows RBTs to evaluate if an activity or aim successfully teaches the desired skills.

(39) (B) Reactionary techniques for unwanted conduct or delayed skill display.

When a client occasionally displays unwanted behavior during skill acquisition sessions, the next best action would be reactionary techniques. These techniques provide a structured response to such behaviors, which ensures that they do not hinder the learning process and that the skill acquisition sessions remain focused and productive.

(40) (B) Use error correction techniques to address the mistake.

According to the essential components of a written skill acquisition plan, the immediate response when a client makes a mistake should be to use error correction techniques. These techniques help address the mistake constructively. The other options suggest that an RBT should ignore the error, reinforce the effort, or change the teaching material entirely. Some of these steps may be appropriate. However, constructive error correction should be the next best step.

(41) (D) Scatterplot data.

If an RBT notices a pattern in the client's behavior related to the time of day, the most effective data collection method is scatterplot data. This method records the occurrence of particular behaviors over an extended period that reveal patterns related to time.

(42) (B) Strategies for skill upkeep and service termination.

When a behavioral therapist plans to fade service hours but maintain therapeutic potential after a client has reached their skill goals, the component of the skill acquisition plan that addresses this process is strategies for skill upkeep and service termination. This component highlights how to reduce service hours correctly while ensuring that the client continues to benefit from the intervention and maintains the acquired skills.

(43) (A) Market research.

Behavioral data's predictive analysis is particularly helpful for market research. First, businesses must understand how people behave in certain situations to target their products and services effectively and align their strategies with consumer behavior patterns. This application of behavioral data allows for more informed decision-making and strategy development in the business context.

(44) (A) Techniques to gather and display data.

Techniques for gathering and displaying data are an essential part of a written skill acquisition plan that allows for a data-driven approach. Data collection is systematic and organized, which enables RBTs to monitor progress, make informed decisions, and adjust teaching strategies based on empirical evidence.

(45) (B) Help the child mentally prepare for the transition.

A visual timer helps the child understand how much time is left for a task and prepares them for the upcoming transition. The visual aspect of the timer is beneficial because it provides a clear and concrete representation of time. Consequently, it reduces anxiety and helps the child mentally prepare for the change in activity. This is particularly helpful for individuals who struggle with abstract concepts of time or sudden changes in routine.

(46) (C) Introduce a fun song related to teeth brushing to make the routine more enjoyable.

The introduction of a fun song related to teeth brushing is an example of a replacement behavior that aligns with ABA principles. This strategy makes the undesired activity (brushing teeth) more enjoyable and can replace the escapist behavior (running away) with a positive and engaging alternative. It addresses the function of the behavior through the alteration of the task's context.

(47) (B) A clear consequence strategy for inappropriate behavior.

A behavior reduction plan must include a clear consequence strategy for inappropriate behavior. This component is essential as it outlines the specific actions that will be taken if the undesired behavior (e.g., banging items on tables) occurs. It helps ensure that the consequences are consistent, predictable, and understood by all parties involved.

(48) (D) Implement deep breathing exercises before transitions.

Deep breathing exercises help the client cope before transitions. This strategy aligns with ABA practices and helps the client remain calm during stressful situations. It also provides the client with a practical and accessible tool to manage their stress and anxiety in other scenarios.

(49) (C) Increase the probability of displaying the demanded behavior and decrease challenging behavior.

Visual objects (e.g., photos, icons, words) can serve as transition strategies to increase the chances that the client will display the demanded behavior and decrease the occurrence of difficult behaviors during transitions. Visual cues provide clear and concrete guidance on what is expected next.

(50) (B) It fulfills the same purpose as the client's original behavior.

When choosing a replacement behavior, it must fulfill the same purpose as the client's original behavior. This ensures that the client's needs are still met but in a more socially acceptable manner.

(51) (D) Provide a faster and easier alternative.

The main purpose of introducing replacement behavior is to provide an action that meets the same need (in this case, getting attention) but is faster, easier, and more socially acceptable. An example is to ask politely instead of screaming. This method encourages the client to adopt the replacement behavior, which is more efficient and yields positive social outcomes.

(52) (C) Data collection procedures to observe and measure the target behavior.

Data collection procedures are a critical component of a behavior reduction plan. These procedures observe, measure, and track the target behavior. They also help evaluate the plan's effectiveness and inform any necessary adjustments.

(53) (C) Teach the child to request a break after a certain period of work.

When the child requests a break, it is considered an appropriate replacement behavior. This behavior serves the same function as when the child escapes the table but in a more acceptable and controlled manner. It allows the child to cope with the demand in a way that can be accommodated and managed within the structure of the task.

(54) (C) Understand and support the components of the plan.

Parents play a vital role in the success of a behavior reduction plan. First, they need to understand and support the plan's components to ensure consistency. Then, they need to align with the strategies and principles outlined in the plan. Ultimately, they can effectively reinforce the desired behaviors and contribute to a cohesive and supportive environment for behavior change.

(55) (C) Socially acceptable and easier than the original behavior.

The key attribute of a replacement behavior is that it should be socially acceptable and easier to perform than the original behavior. This ensures that the client is more likely to adopt the replacement behavior as it meets their needs in a more efficient and appropriate manner. The ease and social acceptability of the replacement behavior increase its effectiveness and the chances of long-term behavior change.

(56) (B) Use a visual timer to provide a clear indication of time left for a task.

A visual timer can serve as a beneficial transition strategy for a client with autism who struggles with changes in routine. The timer provides a clear and concrete representation of the time remaining for a task. This helps the client prepare for the transition and reduces anxiety associated with abrupt changes.

(57) (A) Implement a visual timer or use photo icons.

A visual timer or photo icons can be an effective transition strategy for a client who responds well to visual cues. These visual aids provide a clear and concrete representation of the transition process.

(58) (C) A professional at the BCBA or BCaBA level.

For a client with severe behavior issues, a professional at the BCBA (Board Certified Behavior Analyst) or BCaBA (Board Certified Assistant Behavior Analyst) level is best prepared to write and oversee the behavior reduction plan. These professionals have the necessary training, expertise, and certification to handle complex behaviors and develop individualized intervention plans.

(59) (D) Teach the client to ask politely for the toys.

An effective replacement behavior to assess tangibles is to teach the client to ask politely before they take toys. This replacement behavior fulfills the same function as the original behavior (i.e., to gain access to a desired item) but in a more appropriate manner. It also encourages positive social interactions and respect for others' belongings.

(60) (B) Creates the context for clear communication and ensures procedural fidelity.

When a supervisor states the purpose of supervision, it sets the stage for clear communication between the supervisor and the RBT. It also ensures that both parties understand the objectives and expectations of the supervision process. This clarity helps to create a structured and focused environment conducive to the RBT's professional development and the delivery of high-quality services.

(61) (A) Identify and discuss the causes of insufficient client progress, poor performance, or unethical behavior.

When a supervisor notices that an RBT's client does not make expected progress, it is important to identify and discuss the possible reasons behind this issue. This approach allows for a constructive review of the situation and the development of strategies to address any identified issues. It also ensures the delivery of effective and ethical services to the client.

(62) (B) Feasible supervision capacity based on available time and resources.

Before establishing a supervisory relationship, a supervisor must consider their feasible supervision capacity based on the available time and resources. This consideration ensures that the supervisor can provide adequate attention and support to each RBT. An appropriate capacity fosters a productive and effective supervision environment that benefits the RBTs and their clients.

(63) (C) Supervision content and evaluation of competence for the RBT.

A structured plan that contains supervision content and an evaluation of the RBT's competence is fundamental. This plan sets clear performance expectations and provides a framework to observe and implement behavioral skills training. Moreover, it guides the supervision process and ensures that the RBT receives the necessary guidance and feedback for professional growth.

(64) (B) The supervisor can personally develop a system to document the supervision experience.

According to the BCBA experience standards, supervisors are allowed to develop a personalized system to document their supervision experience. This flexibility acknowledges the unique aspects of each supervisory relationship and allows for a tailored approach to track and reflect on the supervision process.

(65) (A) Monthly.

The RBT must be observed with a client at least once a month. This observation requirement ensures that the supervisor has accurate and up-to-date comprehension of the RBT's interaction with clients and can provide relevant and timely feedback and guidance.

(66) (D) Instruct the RBT based on what the supervisor notices.

The first step is to instruct the RBT based on the supervisor's observations. This initial instruction sets the foundation for the subsequent steps in the supervision process. In essence, it allows the supervisor to address specific areas for improvement and help the RBT enhance their service delivery.

(67) (A) Set goals and provide feedback once the goals have been met.

To motivate trainees, establish clear goals, and give feedback once those goals are met. This approach adopts a sense of accomplishment and progress, which encourages the RBT to continue improving. A supervisor must recognize achievements to maintain the RBT's motivation and commitment to professional growth.

(68) (B) Implement the service plans for the client and assist the advisory team.

The role of the RBT in the service delivery system is to implement the service plans for the client and assist the advisory team. RBTs should directly apply the behavioral interventions under the supervision and direction of higher-level credentials such as BCBA or BCaBA.

(69) (B) Comply with the feedback and work on weak points.

When a supervisor provides feedback, it is vital that the RBT comply with it and actively work on improving any identified weak points. A constructive response to feedback demonstrates commitment to professional development and dedication to providing high-quality services to the clients.

(70) (B) Self-report the situation within thirty days once aware of it.

In the event of legal charges or investigations, the RBT must self-report the situation within thirty days once aware of it. This self-reporting maintains professional and ethical standards and ensures transparency and accountability.

(71) (C) Provide high-quality services that result in client improvement.

The supervisor should highlight that the key purpose of supervision is to provide high-quality services that promote client improvement. This focus on quality and outcome ensures that the supervision process is aligned with the goal of ABA, which is to bring about meaningful and positive change in the client's behavior.

(72) (A) Explore the potential reasons for insufficient client progress.

When a supervisor discusses strategies with the RBT for a client who shows insufficient progress, the focus should be on the exploration of potential reasons for the lack of progress and the discussion of possible solutions. This problem-solving approach promotes a proactive and collaborative effort to address challenges and improve the effectiveness of the intervention.

(73) (D) Develop a structured plan that contains supervision content and an evaluation of the RBT's competence.

For a supervision session to be effective, it is essential to develop a structured plan that includes supervision content and an evaluation of the RBT's competence. This approach ensures that the supervision is focused, comprehensive, and aligned with the RBT's specific needs and professional development goals.

(74) (B) Explore feasible solutions based on available resources.

When an RBT expresses concerns about their workload and client interactions, the supervisor should listen attentively, provide guidance, and explore feasible solutions based on available resources. If the RBT experiences burnout, the measurements taken would be more drastic.

(75) (B) Observe the RBT as they perform the task and keep in mind the previous problems.

After the demonstration, the supervisor's next immediate step is to observe the RBT while they perform the task. This observation allows the supervisor to assess the RBT's application of the instruction and demonstration, which provides a basis for targeted and effective feedback.

(76) (A) At least five hours.

The supervision requirement for an RBT is five percent of the hours they spend during services. Therefore, if an RBT works 100 hours a month, they must be supervised for at least five hours. This requirement ensures that the RBT receives adequate oversight and guidance.

(77) (A) Hold at least two monthly real-time face-to-face meetings.

Effective supervision of an RBT includes at least two monthly real-time face-to-face meetings. These meetings ensure that the supervisor can directly observe and interact with the RBT and provide immediate feedback.

(78) (B) Communicate clear and timely feedback during supervision sessions.

The supervisor must deliver clear and timely feedback during supervision sessions. This practice increases the chances that the RBT understands their performance, recognizes areas for improvement, and receives guidance on how to enhance their skills and service delivery.

(79) (C) Provide instruction on the correct implementation of ABA techniques.

When a supervisor observes that an RBT does not implement ABA techniques properly, the first step is to provide instruction on the correct implementation of these techniques. This step is vital as it addresses the issue directly and gives the RBT the opportunity to learn and correct their methods.

(80) (A) Understand the supervisor's feedback and ask questions.

The main role of the RBT during a supervision session is to listen actively, understand the supervisor's feedback, and ask questions if needed. This receptive and engaged approach allows the RBT to comprehend and apply the feedback to their practice.

(81) (B) Once a month.

The RBT must be observed at least once a month with a client. This required observation ensures that the supervisor accurately comprehends the RBT's interaction with clients and can provide relevant and timely feedback and guidance.

(82) (A) Demonstrate how the problem can be solved.

After instructing the RBT, the supervisor's next step should be to demonstrate how the problem can be solved. This demonstration provides a clear and practical example of the RBT.

(83) (B) Contact the supervisor immediately to address the urgent matter.

If an RBT encounters a situation that requires urgent attention, they should contact the supervisor immediately to resolve the matter. Prompt communication in such cases is vital to resolving issues quickly and effectively.

(84) (A) Accept the feedback and work on areas of improvement.

The expected professional behavior of an RBT in response to feedback is to accept the feedback and work on areas of improvement. This constructive response demonstrates the RBT's commitment to their professional development.

(85) (D) Authorized supervision hours are just general parameters and may be adjusted based on the client's needs.

Authorized supervision hours may need to be adjusted throughout the treatment. This flexibility makes the supervision provided more responsive to the client's individual needs and allows for a more personalized approach to treatment.

Download the Exam Simulator Instructions, Additional Tests and Other Files!

Scan the QR code below with your phone and you will be given a link to Google Drive where you can download the files.

If the QR code does not work for you, please contact us at info@newstonetestprep.com and mention the title of this book.